Radiology and the Law

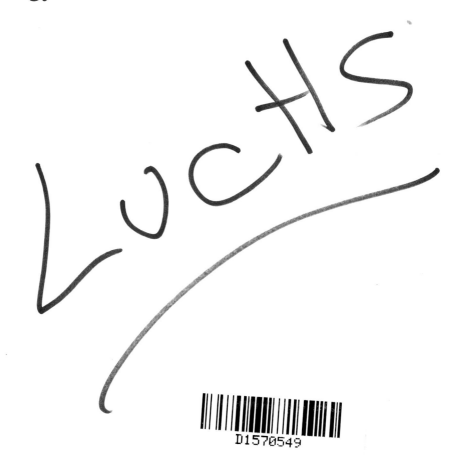

Springer
New York
Berlin
Heidelberg
Hong Kong
London
Milan
Paris
Tokyo

Radiology and the Law
Malpractice and Other Issues

Ronald L. Eisenberg, M.D., J.D.

Chairman, Department of Radiology
Alameda County Medical Center
Oakland, California
Clinical Professor of Radiology
University of California School of Medicine
at Davis and San Francisco

Foreword by John J. Smith, M.D., J.D.

Foreword by William T. Thorwarth, Jr., M.D., F.A.C.R.

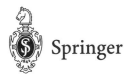 Springer

Ronald L. Eisenberg, M.D., J.D.
Chairman, Department of Radiology
Alameda County Medical Center
Oakland, CA 94602
Clinical Professor of Radiology
University of California School of Medicine
  at San Francisco and Davis
USA
acmcrad@ix.netcom.com

Library of Congress Cataloging-in-Publication Data
Eisenberg, Ronald L.
  Malpractice in radiology / Ronald Eisenberg.
      p. cm.
Includes index.
  ISBN 0-387-40309-4 (softcover : alk. paper)
  1. Radiologists—Malpractice—United States. I. Title.
  KF2910.R333E38 2003
  344.73´04121—dc21   2003052965

ISBN 0-387-40309-4   Printed on acid-free paper.

Printed in the United States of America.

9 8 7 6 5 4 3 2 1   SPIN   10935729

www.springer-ny.com

Springer-Verlag   New York Berlin Heidelberg
A member of BertelsmannSpringer Science+Business Media GmbH

To Zina, Avlana, and Cherina

and

To Leonard Berlin,

Who developed the field of medical-legal radiology

Foreword

Today's radiologist provides clinical service in an environment shaped by a variety of legal and regulatory issues. Whether it is fear of malpractice liability, legal exposure related to electronic imaging, or complying with a wide range of complex government regulations, these issues impact how radiologists perform procedures and studies, report their results, and structure their practices. Despite this impact, most radiologists lack a basic understanding of pertinent legal and regulatory issues, creating a climate of confusion and conflict that benefits neither radiologists nor their patients. Contributing substantially to this environment is the absence of a single, current, readable source of information on radiology and the law.

I can think of no one better qualified than Ron Eisenberg to meet this need. An already accomplished radiologist and author, Dr. Eisenberg took time from his many obligations to attend law school, passing the California Bar Exam in 1996 just two days after receiving his Juris Doctor degree from William Howard Taft University. His clinical experience at a busy county hospital provides a rich real world context with which to identify legal and regulatory issues of concern to the practicing radiologist, his legal background provides the tools to evaluate those issues, and his skills as an author provide the means to effectively communicate that analysis to the radiology community.

The result is the text that follows, addressing the major legal and regulatory issues confronting radiology, all in an organized, thoughtful manner. Topics ranging from tort malpractice and medical liability insurance, to procedure-specific legal considerations, to regulatory issues, and beyond, are discussed in a manner that only Ron Eisenberg can. It is a resource that will well serve the radiology community today, and no doubt in the years to come.

Boston, Massachusetts   *John J. Smith, M.D., J.D.*

Foreword

Every radiologist, indeed every physician, practices today in a climate of legal jeopardy and regulatory oversight. Although this is most commonly perceived in terms of risk of medical malpractice action, the scope of legal issues affecting the practice of radiology far exceeds this one dimension. There are vast libraries dedicated to the continuing education of radiologists regarding new clinical procedures and technological advances. However all of these developments, as well as long-standing established procedures, will be performed under this veil of potential legal scrutiny. Although there is significant literature describing individual components of the legal system relative to radiology, a current comprehensive overview is needed. In this text, Ron Eisenberg, M.D., provides us with a well-organized and practical guide to the multifaceted legal world as it relates to our everyday practices, whether they are private practice or academic.

No radiologist wants to learn firsthand how the legal system works, only to discover that, had the process been better understood, that unpleasant experience could have been totally avoided or one's position could have been substantially improved. None of us would perform a new procedure or practice a new modality without first learning all of the complexities involved. Likewise, we must arm ourselves with a full understanding of those things we can do in our clinical practice, resident oversight, and practice management to minimize our legal and regulatory exposure.

Regarding malpractice, radiologists commonly provide their services with limited or no face-to-face interaction with the patient or the referring physician. This prevents the establishment of a personal relationship that may increase patient tolerance of a poor or unexpected outcome. The communication of imaging findings, as well as the documentation of the results of the procedures we perform, are the radiology "medical record," and the recording and archiving of these form the cornerstone of any retrospective legal analysis. The rapidly evolving technology in the performance, documentation, and communication of radiology services and the ever-expanding volumes of legislation and case law that apply to all aspects of radiology clinical and business practice mandate that radiologists learn the fundamentals and stay current just as we have done with our medical practice. Dr. Eisenberg has provided the launching pad for this career-long journey. Learn and make it a smooth ride.

Hickory, North Carolina

William T. Thorwarth, Jr., M.D.,F.A.C.R.
Chairman, 2003–2005
RSNA Medical Legal Committee
Catawba Radiological Associates

Preface

Few events in a physician's career are as traumatic as a medical malpractice suit. Each year in the United States, it is estimated that the tort system generates nearly one suit for every five physicians overall. Skyrocketing jury awards are a major factor in the substantial increase in malpractice premiums in many states, which have led numerous physicians to retire early, relocate their practices, or consider changing their activities to those with lower risk. Radiologists are among those specialists most frequently involved in litigation. *Radiology and the Law: Malpractice and Other Issues* is designed both to make radiologists aware of how they can become enmeshed in the legal system and to offer ways in which they can decrease their risk of being the focus of a malpractice suit.

The book opens with the basic elements underlying the concept of medical malpractice and a discussion of the anatomy of a medical malpractice suit. It describes the role of the expert witness and standards and practice guidelines at trial, as well as alternative methods of dispute resolution. There is a section analyzing various aspects of professional liability insurance, which unfortunately most radiologists do not consider until after a malpractice suit has been filed against them. This part of the book closes with a discussion of the typical reactions experienced by physicians sued for malpractice and the important role that the radiologist-defendant plays at trial.

The book delves into the cause of interpretive errors and the vexing question of when a missed diagnosis is simply an unfortunate mistake and the point at which it rises to the level of malpractice. Should recognized errors be admitted and, if so, how should they be reported? Once the radiologist has detected all abnormalities and made a reasonable differential diagnosis, it is essential to prepare a written report and properly communicate the imaging findings, especially when they are emergent or "non-urgent but significant." Suggestions are provided as to how radiologists can minimize their legal exposure in these vital areas. There also is the important issue of obtaining informed consent and the two different standards employed by courts in various jurisdictions, as well as the increased medical-legal risks associated with specific examinations, especially breast imaging and interventional procedures. Other topics in this section include whether to use ionic or nonionic contrast material, how to handle the pregnant patient, issues concerning medical devices, and a brief overview of the controversy concerning CT screening studies.

The increasing role of the electronic transmission and storage of images raises a host of new medical-legal issues. *Radiology and the Law: Malpractice and Other Issues* introduces radiologists to licensure and jurisdictional problems relating to teleradiology, confidentiality, and physician–patient–relationship questions with e-mail, and the potential disaster of lost PACS images.

As with all physicians, radiologists are faced with governmental intrusion into their practice. The information in this book provides an overview of such topics as confidentiality and the HIPAA regulations, federal fraud and abuse enforcement, sexual harassment, ERISA, the credentialing and peer review process, and how to handle the radiologist who is affected with a potentially communicable disease or is substance-impaired.

All too often, any discussion of medical malpractice is a depressing experience filled with doom and gloom. Although it addresses the serious implications of a malpractice suit, this text attempts to provide radiologists with at least a glimmer of hope. The adoption of effective risk management techniques decreases the likelihood that a radiologist will fall prey to a malpractice suit, although admittedly this may be the inescapable fate of even the radiologist who has done nothing wrong. If the material in this book spares even one radiologist from the trauma of being the defendant in a malpractice suit, the hours of preparation and writing will have been worth the effort.

I want to gratefully acknowledge my immense debt to Leonard Berlin, whose brilliant series of monthly *Malpractice Issues in Radiology* in the *American Journal of Roentgenology* are the seminal work in the medical-legal literature relating to radiology. In essence, Lenny has almost single-handedly developed the field of medical-legal radiology, making radiologists aware of how the law affects their practices and providing invaluable practical advice for radiologists to minimize their legal exposure. I want to thank John Smith for his encouragement and all the past and current members of the Medical-Legal Committees of the American College of Radiology and the Radiological Society of North America, whose discussions and presentations have refined my knowledge of the subject. Finally, I appreciate the continual support of Rob Albano, Senior Radiology Editor at Springer-Verlag in New York, who asked me to write this book.

Oakland, California   *Ronald L. Eisenberg M.D., J.D.*

Contents

PART II   The Missed Diagnosis: Overview

PART III   Communication and Records

PART IV   Radiology Practice and Specific Procedures

PART V   Electronic Imaging

PART VI   Governmental/Regulatory

Part I
Malpractice Litigation

1
Malpractice

Malpractice is a *tort*, a civil wrong that is not based on the violation of a contract. Tort liability is almost always based on fault—something that was done incorrectly or something that should have been done but was omitted.[1]

The most common theory of liability in medical malpractice is *negligence*, which is defined as "conduct that falls below the standard established by law for the protection of others against unreasonable risk of harm."[2] The negligence cause of action generally requires the plaintiff to establish all of the following four elements:

1. Duty of due care (what should have been done)
2. Breach of this duty (deviation from what should been done)
3. Injury (damages)
4. Causation (injury directly and "legally" caused by the breach of duty)

In effect, what the plaintiff must prove is that the negligent actions of the defendant physician, or a failure to act, was the direct cause of injury (compensable damages) to a patient to whom the physician owed a duty of due care. Each of these four elements presents a legal issue that is argued in a malpractice case.

There is also a "fifth element" that the courts do not discuss but is essential for health care providers to remember—someone must be willing to make a claim. Health care providers who maintain good relationships with their patients before and after untoward incidents are less likely to be sued. Consequently, if a radiologist suspects that an incident possibly amounting to malpractice has occurred, it is vital to notify the person responsible for institutional risk management promptly so that steps can be taken to minimize the chance of a claim being filed.[3]

Duty

The first element that must be proved in any malpractice suit based on negligence is *duty*. This consists of two aspects—that a duty was owed to the person harmed, and the scope of that duty (standard of care).

Existence of a Duty

The common law does not impose a duty on individuals to come to the rescue of persons for whom they have no legal responsibility. Unless otherwise required by state law, a person walking down the street has no *legal* duty to come to the aid of the victim of a heart attack or injury, even though there may be a *moral* obligation to do so, unless (a) the victim is a dependent; (b) the person contributed to the cause of the heart attack or injury; (c) the person owns or operates the premises where the heart attack or injury occurred; or (d) the person has a contractual obligation to come to the victim's aid (such as being a member of a public emergency care team).[4]

The essence of the legal concept of "duty" in medical malpractice is the existence of a physician-patient relationship. This has rarely been an issue in radiology, since virtually all patients who undergo imaging studies are referred by a physician to a specific radiologic facility for identifying the underlying cause of a clinical symptom or physical finding. Once the patient arrives in the radiology department, a physician-patient relationship is established, even though (as is generally the case) the radiologist had no direct contact with the patient.[5] The same principle of duty applies to screening examinations, such as mammography, in which patients may refer themselves for an imaging study.

In most malpractice suits involving radiologists, the existence of a duty is easy to demonstrate. However, as described in the next sections, there are some situations in which a major legal issue may be whether a physician-patient relationship has been established.

Is There a Duty?

"Unofficial" Interpretations[6]

Radiologists may be asked to render unofficial interpretations of studies outside of the formal reading process. This may take the form of a "curbside" (curbstone) consultation, in which a clinician asks the radiologist to "take a quick look at this film" or review a study previously interpreted by another member of the staff. Radiologists have traditionally viewed the giving of curbside consultations as an integral part of daily practice, paying no heed to the possibility that such activity may be placing them in legal jeopardy. The major issue is whether a radiologist providing an informal consultation establishes a physician-patient relationship. Although no appellate cases have dealt specifically with radiologists, various court decisions have focused on nonradiologic curbside consultations. Most state courts have held that physicians who give such informal consultations are immune from malpractice liability by concluding that no physician-patient relationship had been established.[7] However, there are some important exceptions.

In cases absolving physicians from liability for informal consultations, the physicians requesting the opinion generally have relied on themselves rather than on the curbside consultant to make the ultimate decision as to patient treatment. However, the result may be the opposite when the requesting physician relied heavily on the informal consultation in formulating a treatment plan.[8] The legal justification for this view is the analogy to the "duty of a rescuer," the requirement of reasonable care that the law imposes on those who voluntarily undertake to render services to another if they knew that the other person would rely on their actions and consequently forgo other remedies or precautions (e.g., additional tests, referrals).[9] In the radiology context, the key question in the legal analysis may be whether the imaging findings were easily detectable by the requesting physician alone, or whether they were so subtle that they could be seen and interpreted only by a highly skilled radiologist—that is, whether the advice or information given was so specialized that the requesting physician relied on it.

"Although curbside consultations are usually considered as essential means of communication between physicians, some malpractice insurance companies have informed their insureds that such consultations should not be rendered under any circumstances because of the potential medical-legal burden."[10] As one endocrinologist has observed, "It's not in the patient's best interest to respond to curbstone consultations since the consulting physician does not have available to him all of the records, much less the patient, when offering advice…. Curbside consultations should not be rendered under any circumstances."[11]

Nevertheless, the reality of daily practice makes it inevitable that radiologists will be asked to give curbside consultations. Berlin stresses that, whenever possible, the radiologist should attempt to "convert the oral consultation into a formal written report, even offering to do so as a courtesy and without remuneration." Radiologists should stress to physicians seeking informal consultations that "their responses are related to hypothetical questions and not meant to imply a specific diagnosis or [recommended] course of action for a particular patient." If radiologists feel that it is necessary to provide an interpretation based on a brief examination of a radiograph in a rushed manner under less-than-ideal conditions, they "should emphasize that the interpretation is tentative and could be modified when the radiographs are [subsequently] examined under optimal conditions." When a radiologist notes a positive finding in a fresh case, especially if it is subtle and could be missed, it is prudent either to promptly dictate the examination or at least indicate the presence of the abnormality on the requisition or the film. If the radiologist disagrees with a previous reading, it is essential to discuss it with the original interpreter to decide whether to issue an addendum report.

A major problem with curbside consultations is that usually no written documentation of the interpretation is made. Each party may have a different recollection of what was actually said. Even worse, the clinician may note in the patient's chart that a study was reviewed with the radiologist and cite what the radiologist allegedly said, even though the actual interpretation may have been completely different. This is especially critical in situations in which there is high potential exposure (e.g., chest nodule, mammographic lesion, colonic abnormality on barium enema, and prenatal ultrasound). To avoid this situation, with its potential for serious medical-legal consequences, radiologists should document in a written report any informal interpretation that was given. Since this frequently is not a realistic option, radiologists should consider carrying a small notebook in which to briefly document the consultation (patient, referring physician, type of examination, date) and the opinion rendered.

Proctoring

When serving as a proctor observing an interventional procedure, a radiologist probably does not establish a physician-patient relationship. This is based on an analogy to a California appeals court ruling,[12] which held that a surgeon who, on behalf of a hospital and without compensation, volunteered to observe a surgical operation for the sole and express purpose of assessing and reporting on the competence of a surgical candidate for medical staff membership, owed no duty of care to a patient who was injured during the operation.[13] Similarly, a radiologist in a multidepartment teaching conference who recommends surgery for a patient cannot be held liable for malpractice if the patient is subsequently injured during the operative procedure, based in part on the rationale that "the continuing education of its members by the medical profession and the exchange of information between doctors is of great social benefit."[14]

Studies Ordered by a Third Party

In some cases a radiologist may interpret studies at the request of a third party, rather than a referring physician or a patient with whom the radiologist has established a formal physician-patient relationship. The third party may be an employer who requires radiographs to determine eligibility for employment; an insurance company, to determine the insurability of a potential policyholder; a government agency, to assess whether an applicant qualifies for medical disability, Social Security, or workers' compensation benefits; or even a law firm offering free radiographs, to see whether individuals would qualify as potential plaintiffs for inclusion in a class action lawsuit. In all of these situations, the radiologist interpreting the study is retained and compensated by a third party, and the issue arises as to whether the radiologist has established a physician-patient relationship and what is the extent of any duty owed.[15] Clearly, the radiologist is required to use due care in interpreting the examination and communicating the result to the third party that requested the study. But if the radiologist identifies a significant abnormality, is his or her responsibility satisfied by merely communicating the finding to the third party, or is there an independent duty to relay this information directly to the patient? Is the radiologist liable for a failure of communication if the third party does not transmit the abnormal report to the patient, who sustains damages as a result?

Early court decisions ruled that, in the absence of a formal physician-patient relationship, the radiologist has no duty to communicate findings directly to the patient.[16-18] "His duty to use a professional standard of care in making the examination and in preparing the report runs only to the party requesting it.… Even assuming that [the doctor's] conduct fell below the standard of care, it was a breach of duty owed to the [party that retained the doctor], not to [the patient]."[19] However, the modern judicial trend is for courts either to create a physician-patient relationship even where none has traditionally existed, thus greatly expanding the duty of the radiologist to communicate abnormal findings directly to the patient,[20] or to hold that a radiologist can be liable even in the absence of an established physician-patient relationship.[21] The underlying public policy rationale is that a patient undergoing a preemployment or other routine examination "generally assumes that 'No news is good news' and relies on the assumption that any serious condition will be revealed," justifiably believing that, with no report to the contrary, the results of the tests performed must have been negative.[22]

Although some states do not require communication of significant abnormal findings directly to the patient when a study has been performed as part of a contract with a third party, the prudent radiologist should do so, or be certain that the third party contractor has a system in place that reasonably ensures that such information will be communicated to the patient.

Good Samaritan[23]

In emergency situations, do radiologists have a general duty to assist individuals in danger and, if so, are they protected from any adverse consequences of their actions? Although from the moral and ethical point of view, any individual (not just a physician) should provide all possible assistance, under the law in the vast majority of states there is no affirmative legal duty to do so. In the absence of a duty imposed by a physician-patient relationship, no malpractice action can succeed against a physician for failing to provide assistance in an emergency situation. However, for public policy reasons, some courts have implied the existence of such a relationship even if the physician did not intend to create it, as long as the patient had a reasonable expectation of treatment or a belief that the physician has actually begun to provide it. Merely being on an airplane when a fellow passenger becomes ill would not create a legal duty for a physician to offer assistance. However, a court probably would construe the existence of a duty if a radiologist failed to respond to a patient having an anaphylactic reaction, even if he or she had not actually administered the intravenous contrast material, as long as the patient was registered in the department where the radiologist was working. Moreover, the existence of a valid physician-patient relationship may result from judicial interpretation of specific provisions in a hospital's medical staff bylaws, to which all physicians agree to abide as a requirement of obtaining and retaining privileges.

A survey of internists detailed various reasons why they would not offer care in an emergency situation. These included the fear of contracting an infectious disease, lack of comfort with their acute medical care skills, and the belief that it was not their responsibility to help. Almost 20% cited the fear of legal liability. Indeed, the fear of lawsuits filed by ungrateful emergency victims against their voluntary benefactors was the underlying reason for all states to enact Good Samaritan laws. These provide that, as long as they have no previous knowledge of the illness or injury and do not accept payment for the emergency aid given, physicians have no exposure for malpractice liability for complications of their efforts unless there is gross negligence or a lack of good faith. Of course, this does not prevent a plaintiff from filing a lawsuit alleging either that the physician was not acting as a Good Samaritan or that the treatment rendered constituted "willful, wanton, or gross negligence." Conceivably, if a provision in the hospital bylaws requires that a physician respond to in-hospital emergencies, a plaintiff could argue that the physician had a preexisting duty to do so (i.e., was not acting as a Good Samaritan), and thus only the standard principles of negligence would apply.

Berlin emphasizes that "whether a radiologist or other physician can even be brought before a jury for alleged malpractice resulting from refusal to render emergency treatment is a decision that is made by a judge, presumably only on the basis of law." However, if a trial ensues, "a jury of laypersons is not likely to view with great enthusiasm or sympathy statements offered by the defendant radiologist that he or she refused to render care to a patient who was in immediate danger of serious injury or death because the defendant 'wasn't qualified,' 'didn't think it was his or her responsibility,' 'didn't want to get involved,' or 'was afraid of being sued.'"

Other Duties

Duty to Refer

A *duty to refer* generally applies when a radiologist is unable to provide satisfactory care to a patient due to a limitation of personal knowledge or experience or the unavailability of equipment to perform the clinically appropriate examination. In the most common situation, it is necessary to consult a specialist because the case is clearly outside the limits of a generalist's skill or knowledge. In a nonradiologic case, a general practitioner was held liable for complications relating to the treatment of a fracture when it was shown that the physician had not read any text on the setting of fractures since his graduation from medical school more than 30 years earlier. It should be noted that the duty to keep knowledge current is reasonably flexible—physicians are not required to keep up-to-date on all phases of medical progress, but rather only with respect to the types of cases that they agree to undertake.[24] A radiologist who does not have the skill or experience to interpret a certain type of examination or perform a specific interventional procedure has a duty to refer the patient to a colleague who possesses these attributes.

When a certain type of study cannot properly be done with existing equipment, there is a duty to refer the patient to an institution that maintains such equipment and can perform the procedure correctly. Many institutions cannot afford to offer every type of procedure (and expertise) for their patient population. However, the mere fact that some facilities have more advanced equipment than others does not necessarily imply that the latter are incapable of providing appropriate care. In some situations, various approaches to a clinical problem may be equally valid in terms of efficacy. For example, although magnetic resonance (MR) and computed tomography (CT) angiography are increasingly employed to evaluate noninvasively vascular anatomy and function, some reports have suggested limitations of these procedures. Because catheter arteriography is an acceptable means of studying vascular anatomy under most circumstances, a facility that does not provide MR or CT angiography need not necessarily refer the patient to another institution, especially if there is a high likelihood that the patient may require an interventional procedure in which contemporaneous correction by angioplasty is afforded with an arteriographic study when the catheter in place can be readily exchanged for a balloon dilatation catheter. Of course, as part of the informed consent process, the radiologist would have to provide a comprehensive discussion of the noninvasive alternative, though he or she would be justified in expressing a preference for arteriography (as long as the information is not misrepresented to the patient). However, the situation is entirely different if another type of study, not offered at the institution, is clearly preferable but not discussed because of the costs involved. Although courts have ruled that costs may be considered in the management of patients, cost considerations will not excuse the liability of a physician if substandard care is rendered.[25]

Duty to Refuse to Perform a Not-Indicated Procedure

Most patients for diagnostic or interventional imaging procedures are referred to the radiologist by a treating physician. Radiologists generally defer to the judgment of referring clinicians as to whether a study is indicated. However, as an independent physician and not the agent of the referring clinician, it is the radiologist who has the ultimate responsibility for assuring the appropriateness and proper performance of the procedure. Consequently, the radiologist has a duty to decline to comply with a request for a not-indicated diagnostic examination or an inappropriate interventional study that would violate the standard of reasonable care. For example, in the setting of a patient with acute flank pain suggestive of ureteral stone, a radiologist should refuse a urologist's request for a excretory urogram and instead insist that the patient receive a noncontrast CT, which provides superior diagnostic accuracy without the risk of a contrast reaction. Similarly, a radiologist should decline to perform a pulmonary arteriogram instead of CT as the initial procedure in a patient with suspected pulmonary embolism. Interventional radiologists should not agree to perform procedures unless they have sufficient surgical backup, lest they be held liable for the nonavailability of a physician capable of treating a reasonably foreseeable complication. In all of these cases, the radiologist must call the physician who has referred the patient and explain the reasoning behind his or her refusal to comply with the request. If the referring clinician remains adamant that the procedure be performed as ordered, the radiologist should be resolute and politely suggest that the referring clinician may wish to see whether another facility would accede to the request. Once the patient has effectively been referred back to the treating physician pursuant to this discussion, the duty of the radiologist to the patient has terminated.[26]

Scope of the Duty (Standard of Care)

Once the existence of a physician-patient relationship has been established, the radiologist owes that patient a duty to act as a reasonably prudent radiologist would have done in similar circumstances, "possessing and exercising that degree of reasonable skill and knowledge which is ordinarily possessed by other members of the profession."[27] Individuals who have acquired special competence are held to a standard commensurate with their superior knowledge or skills,[28] so that a radiologist is held to the minimum standards of that specialty, which obviously are higher than those of physicians at large. Until relatively recently, physicians and other professionals were held to the standard of care prevailing in the community in which they practiced (or similar locale).[29] This rule was designed to avoid finding rural physicians liable for not following the practices of urban medical centers. The requirement that experts testifying on the standard of care had to be from the same or similar communities sometimes made it difficult to obtain expert testimony.[30] However, as professional education has become more uniform nationally, most courts have abolished the "local standards" rule and replaced it with a national standard of care for nationally certified specialists.[31,32] Nevertheless, the jury is usually permitted to consider the expert's degree of familiarity with the community in deciding what weight to give the testimony.[33]

In a malpractice suit, the jury determines whether the radiologist met the standard of care based on one or more of the following: (a) expert testimony, (b) common sense, and (c) written standards.[34] The plaintiff generally must present the testimony of expert witnesses to establish the standard of care required of a radiologist and to demonstrate that the defendant fell below that standard. Because the plaintiff may introduce the radiologist's out-of-court statements as an admission, it is important to be careful what one says (or writes) after an incident.[35] Nontechnical aspects of care can be proven by nonexperts. When the defendant's conduct was so egregious and obvious that a layperson using common sense could identify the breach of duty (e.g., amputating the wrong leg), no expert testimony is needed.[36] In the radiology arena, some courts have ruled that failure to use restraints to prevent a disoriented patient from falling off an x-ray table was an issue of routine, nontechnical care.[37]

A third method for determining the scope of duty is an assessment of written standards, such as licensure regulations, accreditation standards, and institutional rules. Depending on the jurisdiction,[38] these can be considered as (a) evidence the jury can consider in determining the standard of care without any supporting expert testimony[39]; (b) evidence the jury can consider in determining the standard of care, but only if there is also expert testimony confirming that the published standard states the actual standard of care[40]; or (c) presumptive evidence of the standard of care that the jury must accept unless the defendant can prove otherwise.[41] Radiologists must be aware of and act in compliance with all institutional rules and policies referable to their area of practice. If the rules are impossible to follow, steps should be taken to modify them instead of ignoring them. Eliminating all institutional rules is not a viable solution, because the failure to adopt necessary rules can itself be a violation of the standard of care. Thus not having procedures for determining whether angiographic catheters have been recalled could be a mere administrative issue that does not require expert testimony.[42]

The development of medical practice guidelines, practice parameters, clinical protocols, and other guidelines for clinical decision making have complicated the issue of written standards. For the role of the numerous standards issued by the American College of Radiology in malpractice suits, see page 30.

Infrequently, statutes or governmental regulations can be used to establish the standard of care. When a law requires an action in order to benefit other individuals or forbids an action to protect others, a violation is generally considered *negligence per se*. An individual who is harmed by such a violation need prove only that (a) the law is intended to benefit the class of persons of which the individual is a member; (b) the law was violated; (c) the injury is of the type that the law was intended to prevent; and (d) the injury was caused by the violation. As an example, if a radiologist performs a biopsy with a needle suspected of not being sterile, requiring postponement of other therapy and immediate treatment to prevent infection from the needle, the hospital may be found liable for the injuries because of failure to comply with a hospital licensing regulation requiring segregation of sterile and nonsterile needles, since this was the type of patient and harm the regulation was designed to address.[43]

Respected Minority Rule

Proving what constitutes the standard of care can be difficult when there are two or more professionally accepted approaches to a given clinical situation. This gives rise to the concept of the *respected minority* or *two schools of thought rule*. In brief, radiologists are precluded from liability if they follow the approach used by a considerable number of respected physicians in the specialty, since there is no legal duty to follow the majority approach.[44] However, since part of the informed consent process (see page 139) is to disclose alternative treatments, radiologists generally should discuss with the patient the approach used by the majority before pursuing a minority approach. Indeed, failure to disclose the alternative majority approach could result in liability under the informed consent doctrine.[45]

Breach of Duty

After the existence and scope of the duty have been demonstrated, the plaintiff in a malpractice suit based on negligence must prove that the defendant committed a breach of that duty. The physician must have deviated from the standard of care—either doing something that should not have been done (commission), or failing to do something that should have been done (omission). The expert witness is asked whether, in his or her opinion, the actions of the defendant breached the standard of a care "to a reasonable medical certainty," which effectively means "more likely than not."

Injury (Damages)

The third element of proof required of the plaintiff in a malpractice action based on negligence is the demonstration of some physical, financial, or emotional injury that was caused by the physician's deviation for the standard of care. The existence of the injury is generally evident at the time of the suit, though there may still be some disagreement concerning its dollar value. *Special damages* are awarded to the successful plaintiff-patient for expenses that are directly related and actual consequences of the injury suffered. Examples of special damages are the plaintiff's out-of-pocket losses, such as medical expenses, lost wages, and costs of rehabilitation. *General damages* are those that the law presumes to accumulate from the natural consequences of the negligent act. These intangible damages include pain and suffering, disfigurement, and interference with ordinary enjoyment of life. Courts recognize that mental and emotional distress can be just as real as physical pain. In most courts, however, negligently inflicted emotional injuries are compensated only if there is also proof of physical injury. Nevertheless, a few states (such as California) permit compensation to those who witness injury to close relatives. Some even allow compensation to those who claim emotional injury from possible exposure to the human immunodeficiency virus (HIV) without any evidence of their having been infected.

Punitive or *exemplary damages* are financial compensation to plaintiffs over and above their actual losses or expenses. Although frequently alleged in medical malpractice cases, they are rarely awarded. The purpose of punitive damages is to punish outrageous acts, which need not be intentional but are of such a nature that they exhibit incompetent treatment or a reckless disregard for the well-being of the patient. Examples include physicians who practice while under the influence of alcohol or drugs or who fail to respond to repeated calls to come to the hospital to care for their patients.

Causation

The breach of duty must be proved to have legally caused the injury. Although this often seems obvious, causation is often the most difficult element to prove in a negligence lawsuit. For example, if a patient dies following an interventional radiologic procedure that was performed in a negligent manner, the plaintiff must demonstrate a substantial likelihood that the patient would have lived if the procedure had been performed properly. Patients with advanced malignancy often have difficulty pressing malpractice claims because their underlying conditions are probably terminal. To make it easier for such plaintiffs to win their suits, some courts have adopted a new standard of causation termed the *loss of chance* of recovery. Under this standard, the plaintiff must show only that the defendant's breach of the standard of care led to a loss of chance of recovery or survival, rather than that the breach caused the injury.[46] Initially, this standard of causation required a showing of a loss of chance of recovery or survival of greater than 50%.[47] In recent years, however, some courts have allowed claims to proceed in cases where the loss of chance of recovery was substantially less, even as low as 10%.[48]

At times, an "intervening act" that occurred *after* the defendant's negligent act may break the chain of causation. These are often termed "superseding causes," since they supersede (*cancel*) the defendant's liability.[49] Criminal or tortuous acts or gross negligence by third persons, as well as bizarre or highly unusual intervening causes, have been held to be superseding when they produce an unforeseeable result, one that is different from the threat that made the defendant's conduct negligent. For example, a physician whose negligence resulted in a patient's being hospitalized would not be liable for the death of that patient if murdered by a crazed gunman.

Res Ipsa Loquitur

An exception to the requirement that the four elements be proved to establish negligence is the doctrine of *res ipsa loquitur* ("the thing speaks for itself"). This doctrine was created in an 1863 case in which a barrel flying out of an upper story window smashed into a pedestrian and caused substantial injury. When the pedestrian attempted to sue the building owner, he could not discover what went wrong in the building and thus would have lost his case had the court not ruled that there should be liability when someone had clearly done something wrong. The doctrine of *res ipsa loquitur* applies when the following elements can be proven: (a) the accident is of a kind that does not happen without negligence; (b) the apparent cause was in the exclusive control of the defendant; (c) the person injured could not have contributed to the damages; (d) evidence of the true cause is inaccessible to the person suing; and (e) the fact of the injury is evident. Courts have frequently applied this rule to two types of malpractice cases—sponges and other foreign objects unintentionally left in the body, and injuries to parts of the body distant from the site of treatment.[50] Thus a radiologist could be liable for negligence if a portion of a catheter is left in a patient after an angiogram or if a patient suffers nerve damage to the hand after a long interventional procedure involving the leg or abdomen. Nevertheless, liability is not automatic in such cases, for the defendant is permitted to explain why the injury was not the result of negligence (i.e., the burden of proof shifts from the plaintiff to the defendant, who must rebut the presumption of negligence).[51]

Defenses and Limitations to a Malpractice Suit

Statute of Limitations

Because of the belief that the passage of time makes defending law suits unreasonably burdensome, all states have passed legislation limiting the filing of malpractice suits to a specified time period after the alleged act of malpractice occurred. These statutes of limitations generally range from 2 to 3 years and, depending on the state, may begin at the time (a) the incident occurred, (b) the injury was discovered, (c) the cause of the injury was or should have been discovered, or (d) the patient stopped receiving care from the negligent provider. Most states will extend, or "toll," the running time prescribed in the statute if the injured patient is a minor, legally or mentally incompetent, or incarcerated. For injuries to children, in many states the time period for the statute of limitations does not start until they become adults, so that suits arising out of the care of newborns may be filed 18 or more years later.[52] Fraudulent concealment by a physician of any medical acts or errors will also extend the statutory period during which a malpractice suit can be filed.[53,54]

The statutory period varies among the states because of different opinions concerning the underlying purpose of the law. A longer statute of limitations is perceived to be of benefit to injured patients, who might be unable to discover their injuries quickly enough. Moreover, some argue that it might deter physicians from committing malpractice if they realize that they will be forced to pay for their negligent care regardless of when it becomes evident. Conversely, a shorter statute of limitations is generally viewed as beneficial to the defendant physician, who otherwise might be inappropriately held liable on the basis of stale evidence and hindsight medical testimony. However, a shorter statute runs the risk of encouraging physicians to conceal their negligent acts because of the likelihood that evidence of malpractice will not be discovered during that period. Some maintain that shortening the statute of limitations is of value because it encourages patients who are injured by malpractice to act decisively, rehabilitate themselves, and generally "get on with their lives."[55]

Continuum of Care Doctrine

For public policy reasons, courts are reluctant to apply the statute of limitations too strictly lest it have a chilling effect on the access of an injured patient to the courtroom. One theory accepted in about 40% of states is the *continuum of care* doctrine, which tolls the commencement of the statute of limitations in cases in which a physician provides continuing care over a period of time to a particular patient for a specific injury or illness until the treatment of the condition has ended or the relationship between the doctor and patient is terminated, regardless of the actual time of occurrence of the alleged act of negligence. This legal concept is based on the premise that a physician has a continuing obligation to correct an error made during the course of treatment, and that failure to do so constitutes continuing negligence. Originally, the continuum of care doctrine was applied only to physicians involved in direct patient care. However, in certain states it has been extended to consulting physicians such as radiologists, who, although not providing direct continuing care to patients, nevertheless provide diagnostic opinions on which primary care physicians base ongoing treatment decisions. Some courts have held that because the standard of care requires radiologists to compare current imaging studies with previous ones, radiologists are effectively "reinterpreting" all previous radiographs whenever they interpret new studies. Under this theory, the statute of limitations begins to run when the radiologist interprets the most recent follow-up examination, rather than on the date on which the initial studies were obtained. Other courts have ruled that when radiologists maintain no contact with a patient aside from rendering a diagnosis imparted directly to the treating physician, the performance of each diagnosis is complete and discrete and does not constitute continuous treatment, even if on successive occasions the radiologist compared prior studies with the most recent one.[56]

Release

When a claim is settled, the claimant usually signs a release that generally bars a future malpractice suit based on the same incident. Sometimes the release of one defendant, such as a hospital, will also release other defendants, such as radiologists and other physicians (and vice versa). However, the various courts are split on this issue. Releases on behalf of minors are often later attacked by the minors when the reach maturity. Therefore, special attention must be focused on complying with state requirements, which often require court approval of the settlement, to ensure that such releases are legally binding.[57]

Exculpatory Contract

The patient may sign a contract agreeing not to sue, or to limit the amount of the suit, before care is provided. However, in the context of providing health care services, courts have consistently refused to enforce such contracts on the grounds that they are against public policy.[58]

Contributory/Comparative Negligence

Each person has a duty to exercise due care to avoid his own injury at the hands of another. Failure to do what a reasonable person would have done to protect himself under the same or similar circumstances, if it played a role in his sustaining his injury, is termed *contributory negligence* and may preclude or at least reduce the responsibility of the physician for the damage. Examples of contributory negligence include (a) failure of the patient to follow clear orders or return for routine follow-up care; (b) failure of the patient to seek emergency follow-up care when he or she knows or suspects a problem; and (c) the deliberate giving of false information that leads to an otherwise reasonable action on the part of the physician. The success of this defense depends in large measure on the intelligence and degree of orientation of the patient. Therefore, because a patient who seems too confused to follow orders cannot be relied upon to do so, the defense of contributory negligence would not be successful in such a situation.[59]

Under common law, a plaintiff's contributory negligence was an absolute and complete bar to any recovery for the negligence of the defendant. This harsh "all-or-nothing" rule was true regardless of how slight the negligence of the plaintiff was as compared to that of the defendant.[60]

The vast majority of states have rejected this all-or-nothing approach and adopted a fairer system that attempts to apportion damages between the plaintiff and the defendant according to their relative degree of fault (*comparative negligence*). California and New York utilize a "pure" comparative negligence, which allows the plaintiff to recover a percentage of her damages even when her own negligence exceeds that of the defendant. Thus if the jury determines that the plaintiff was 80% at fault, she could still recover 20% of her damages.[61] Most states, however, recognize only "partial" comparative negligence and deny any recovery to a plaintiff whose own negligence exceeds some threshold level. For example, if the standard is "equals or is greater than the defendant," the plaintiff cannot recover if the negligence is apportioned 50-50 (a common occurrence since juries often regard the negligence of both sides as about the same).[62]

Damage Caps

During an economically unstable period during the mid-1970s, the largest liability carrier in California decided to exit the liability underwriting business, leaving physicians frantically searching for some carrier willing to provide coverage. This led to legislative enactment of the Medical Injury Compensation Reform Act (MICRA) of 1975, which limited trial court decisions of special awards for pain and suffering to a maximum of $250,000. Other states also have enacted statutory limits on the amount that can be awarded in malpractice suits. However, in several states such "tort reform" legislation has been defeated by the intense opposition of state and national trial lawyer associations, whose political contributions are among the highest of any organization.[63] Courts have disagreed on the constitutionality of such limits.[64] For example, the Illinois Supreme Court has declared damage caps to be a violation of the constitutional requirement of equal protection because it could find no rational justification for treating those injured by medical malpractice differently from those injured by other means.[65,66] Conversely, the Indiana Supreme Court ruled that damage caps were constitutional because the need for a risk-spreading mechanism to assure the continued availability of health services provided a rational justification.[67] Critics have complained that the fixed limits for pain and suffering are too low—the California limit has not changed in more than 20 years—and thus there may be a push to make future adjustments in the damage cap in this and other states to account for inflation.[68]

Endnotes

1 Miller RD, Hutton RC. *Problems in Health Care Law, 8th ed.* Gaithersburg (MD), Aspen, 2000, pg. 361.
2 Restatement (Second) of Torts #282 (1965).
3 Miller RD, Hutton RC. *Problems in Health Care Law, 8th ed.* Gaithersburg (MD), Aspen, 2000, pg.
4 Ibid., 366.

5 Howard ML. Physician-patient relationship. In: Sanbar SS, Gibofsky A, Friestone MH, et al (eds). *Legal Medicine, 5th ed.* St. Louis, Mosby, 2001, pgs 235–244.

6 Berlin L. Curbstone consultations. *AJR* 2000;178:1351–1359.

7 *Reynolds v Decatur Memorial Hospital*, 277 3d80 (Ill App 1996).

8 *Diggs v Arizona Cardiologist, Ltd.*, Ariz Ct. App. No. 1 CA-CV 99-0508 (8/8/2000).

9 Hendel T. Informal consultations: do new risks exist with this age-old tradition? *Medical Practice Management*, May–June 2002:308–311.

10 Block MB. Curbside consultations and malpractice policies. (letter) *JAMA* 1999;281:899; cited in footnote 6.

11 Block MB. Personal communication, cited in footnote 6.

12 *Clarke v Hoek*, 174 ed 208 (Cal App 1985).

13 Berlin L. The importance of patient registration and processing. *AJR* 1997;169:1483–1486.

14 *Rainer v Grossman*, 31 3d539 (Cal App 1973).

15 Berlin L. Are radiologists contracted by third parties to interpret radiographs liable for not communicating results directly to patients? *AJR* 2002;178:27–33.

16 *Adams v Harron*, LEXIS 21937 (US 4th Cir 1999).

17 *Beaman v Helton & Helton*, 573 So2d 776 (Miss 1990).

18 *Adams v Harron*, LEXIS 21937 (US 4th Cir 1999).

19 *Hafner v Beck*, 916 P2d 1105 (Ariz App 1995).

20 Berlin L. Are radiologists contracted by third parties to interpret radiographs liable for not communicating results directly to patients? *AJR* 2002;178:27–33.

21 *Meena v Wilburn*, 603 So2d 866 (Miss 1992).

22 *Betesh v United States of America*, 400 F Supp 238 (US Dist DC 1974).

23 Berlin L. The good samaritan. *AJR* 2001;177:529–534.

24 Eisenberg RL. Obstetrical ultrasonography: ectopic pregnancy. In: *Risk Management: Test and Syllabus*. Reston, VA: American College of Radiology, 1999:29–35.

25 Brenner RJ. Angiographic interventional procedures. In: *Risk Management: Test and Syllabus*. Reston, VA: American College of Radiology, 1999:13–17.

26 Ibid.

27 *Ritchie v. West*, 23 Ill 329 (1860); cited in Berlin L. Does the missed radiographic diagnosis constitute malpractice? *Radiology* 1977;123:523–527.

28 Restatement (Second) of Torts #289 (b).

29 *Tallbull v Whitney*, 564 P.2d 162 (Mont. 1977).

30 Miller RD, Hutton RC. *Problems in Health Care Law, 8th ed.* Gaithersburg (MD), Aspen, 2000, pg. 369.

31 *Robbins v Footer*, 553 F.2d 123 (D.C. Cir 1977).

32 *Morrsion v MacNamara*, 407 A.2d 555 (D.C. 1979).

33 Miller RD, Hutton RC. *Problems in Health Care Law, 8th ed.* Gaithersburg (MD), Aspen, 2000, pg. 369.

34 Ibid., 366.

35 *Brookover v Mary Hitchcock Memorial Hospital*, 893 F.2d 411 (1st Cir 1990).

36 *Heimer v Privratsky*, 434 N.W. 2d 357 (N.D. 1989).

37 *Cockerton v Mercy Hospital Medical Center*, 490 N.W.2d 856 (Iowa Ct App 1992).

38 Miller RD, Hutton RC. *Problems in Health Care Law, 8th ed.* Gaithersburg (MD), Aspen, 2000, pg. 367.

39 *Peacock v Samaritan Health Services*, 159 Ariz 123, 765 P.2d 525 (Ct. App 1988).

40 *Van Iperen v Van Bramer*, 392 N.W.2d 480 (Iowa 1986).

41 *Hastings v Baton Rouge General Hospital*, 498 So.2d 713 (La. 1986).

42 Miller RD, Hutton RC. *Problems in Health Care Law, 8th ed.* Gaithersburg (MD), Aspen, 2000, pg. 368.

43 Ibid., 368–369.

44 *Jones v Chidester*, 531 Pa. 31, 610 A.2d 964 (1992).

45 Miller RD, Hutton RC. *Problems in Health Care Law, 8th ed.* Gaithersburg (MD), Aspen, 2000, pg. 369.

46 Howard ML. Physician as defendant in medical malpractice. In: Sanbar SS, Gibofsky A, Firestone MH, et al (eds). *Legal Medicine, 5th ed.* St. Louis, Mosby, 2001, pgs 85–86.

47 *Wallace v St. Francis Hospital & Medical Center*, 44 Conn App 257, 688 A.2d 352 (1997).

48 *Wendland v Sparks*, 574 N.W.2d 327 (Iowa 1998).

49 Restatement (Second) of Torts #440 (1965).

50 Miller RD, Hutton RC. *Problems in Health Care Law, 8th ed.* Gaithersburg (MD), Aspen, 2000, pg. 372.

51 *Mulkey v Tubb*, 535 So.2d 1294 (La. Ct App 1988).

52 Miller RD, Hutton RC. *Problems in Health Care Law, 8th ed.* Gaithersburg (MD), Aspen, 2000, pg. 373.

53 *Keithley v St. Joseph's Hospital*, 698 P2d 435 (N Mex App 1984).

54 *Muller v Thuat*, 430 NW2d 884 (Neb 1988).

55 Bovbjert RR, Schumm JM. Judicial policy and quantitative research: Indiana's statute of limitations for medical practitioners. *Indiana Law Rev* 1998;31:1051–1085.

56 Berlin L. Statute of limitations and the continuum of care doctrine. *AJR* 2001;177: 1011–1016.

57 Ibid., 374.

58 Ibid., 375.

59 Ibid., 376.

60 Restatement (Second) of Torts #467 (1965).

61 *Li v Yellow Cab Co. of California*, 532 P.2d 1226 (Cal. 1975).

62 *Bevan v Vassar Farms, Inc.*, 793 P.2d 711 (Idaho 1990).

63 Brenner RJ. The malpractice crisis, 2002: here we go again. *Imaging Economics*, October 2002:6–12.

64 Miller RD, Hutton RC. *Problems in Health Care Law, 8th ed.* Gaithersburg (MD), Aspen, 2000, pg. 377.

65 *Wright v Central DePage Hospital Association*, 63 Ill. 2d 313, 347 N.E.2d 736 (1976).

66 *Best v Taylor Machine Works Co.*, 179 Ill. 2d 367, 689 N.E. 2d 1057 (1997).

67 *Johnson v St. Vincent Hospital*, 273 Ind. 374, 404 N.E. 2d 585 (1980).

68 Brenner RJ. The malpractice crisis, 2002: here we go again. *Imaging Economics*, October 2002:6–12.

2
Vicarious Liability

An employer is vicariously liable for any tortuous acts committed by an employee within the scope of employment. Known legally as *respondeat superior* (literally, "let the person higher up answer"), the Latin term derives historically from the liability of a servant that was imputed to the master. In the contemporary medical setting, it refers to the liability relationships among staff physicians and nurses, technologists, and residents, or between hospitals and physicians. It is important to remember that staff radiologists may be held liable for the actions of their technologists or residents, even though their own conduct may have been completely blameless.

The concept of vicarious liability is predicated on the belief that an employer who assigns specific duties to employees and will gain financial benefits from their actions should be responsible for any harm resulting from such actions. Vicarious liability applies even if the tortuous acts were not committed in the presence of the employer, who thus had no actual ability to control the employee's conduct. Ironically, an employer may be held liable for torts committed by an employee who is immune from liability. For example, if a husband negligently injures his wife at work, the wife may hold the employer vicariously liable, even if she cannot maintain an action directly against her husband because of interspousal immunity.

Vicarious liability is based on the concept of the "deep pocket" (see page 67). According to this theory, compensation for accidents arising directly or indirectly out of an enterprise should be paid by the entrepreneur as a "cost of doing business." Moreover, employees are often "judgment proof," since they do not have sufficient assets to pay a substantial damage award. Unlike employers, who virtually always carry liability insurance against work-related accidents, employees infrequently have such coverage.

For vicarious liability to exist, the employee must have acted "within the scope of employment." This means that the negligent act occurred while the employee was intending to further the employer's business purpose, even if the means the employee chose were indirect, misguided, or even expressly forbidden by the employer. An employee is deemed to be within the scope of business if any deviation (i.e., going for a personal purpose) is considered to be "reasonably foreseeable," such as going to lunch, to the bathroom, or outside the department to smoke.

In general, intentional, nonnegligent torts, such as assault, battery, and false imprisonment, do not create vicarious liability for the employer. Therefore, if an employee violently dislikes a patient/customer, gets into an argument, and strikes him or her, most courts would hold that the employer is not liable. However, a growing minority would disagree, considering that since the tort really arose out of the employment, the employer should be liable.

Employees Versus Independent Contractors

The distinction between employees and independent contractors has traditionally been the critical distinction that determines whether the employer can be held vicariously liable. The key issue is the degree of control that the hirer exerts over the physical details of the work; the greater the control, the more likely the hiree would be considered an employee and the employer vicariously liable. With independent contractors, unlike employees, the employer has no right to control the manner in which the contract is performed.

Liability for Acts of Technologists

In most hospitals and clinics, radiology technologists are employed by the facility and radiologists are independent contractors. Under such an arrangement, the hospital or clinic that pays the salary of the radiology technologists assumes sole legal liability for their negligent acts. Nevertheless, according to a legal doctrine known as the *borrowed servant* rule, vicarious liability may extend to a radiologist who does not employ a technologist, but acquires the same right of supervisory control over the technologist (employee) as was possessed by the lending employer (hospital).[1] Indeed, in some states, when an employer (hospital) delegates its right to direct and control the activities of an employee (technologist) to an independent staff physician (radiologist) who assumes responsibility, the radiologist may be liable for the acts of the technologist and the hospital absolved from liability. However, courts in many states do not apply the borrowed servant doctrine when an employee continues to receive substantial direction from the hospital through its policies and rules. The overall trend appears to be the adoption of a *dual servant* doctrine, under which both the physician and the hospital are vicariously liable for the acts of the employee.[2] The radiologist also may be subjected to vicarious liability under the concept of *apparent* or *ostensible agency*, if it can be shown that that the actions or statements of the radiologist would lead the reasonably prudent person to believe that the technologist was controlled by the radiologist.[3]

There are three basic ways in which radiologists can be vicariously liable for injuries related to the negligence of their technologists. *Slip and fall* is the catchall term applied to lawsuits filed by patients who claim to have been injured as a result of falling off examination tables, gurneys, or chairs; slipping on floors or tripping over furniture; or being accidentally struck by parts of imaging equipment. A classic example is the patient who falls from the x-ray table because he or she was not properly secured with safety straps by the technologist while moving from the horizontal to the vertical position. Another is the trauma patient who becomes quadriplegic after the technologist removes a cervical collar. In both of these cases, radiologists may be named as codefendants even though they were not present when the injury occurred.[4]

Patient injuries can result from technologists' violating departmental policies. For example, the radiologist may perform a procedure that would have been canceled had the technologist informed the radiologist that the patient thought she might be pregnant. If the patient later delivers a child with congenital anomalies, the radiologist may be named in a resulting malpractice suit. Similarly, a technologist may fail to carry out departmental policy by informing the radiologist about a patient's history of contrast allergy, leading to a severe reaction when high-osmolarity contrast rather than nonionic contrast was administered. At times, radiologists may risk vicarious liability when the technologist is following a direct order. This may occur when the technologist overinflates the retention cuff of an enema tip, resulting in a perforated rectum, or prematurely releases pressure on the groin of a patient who has undergone arteriography, producing a large hematoma. Under the previous and similar scenarios, plaintiffs' attorneys may be particularly inclined to include a radiologist as a codefendant with a hospital or clinic if it is unclear which of the parties should be vicariously liable, or if it is uncertain whether the hospital or clinic has sufficient insurance coverage or other financial resources to pay a high damage award.[5]

Court rulings vary widely on the issue of whether physicians are subject to vicarious liability for the negligent actions of their nurses and technologists. Independent-contractor radiologists based in hospitals or clinics should seek legal advice as to ways to modify their written contracts so as to minimize their risk of incurring vicarious liability. In addition, they should determine which departmental policies and procedures have been developed by and are directly related to the health care facility, and which have been formulated or approved by the radiologists. However, the key to decreasing exposure for vicarious liability is for radiologists to exercise their best judgment in determining how much direct supervision of technologists is required for specific imaging examinations or in the daily operation of a health care facility.[6]

When both the technologist and the radiologist are employees of the same hospital or clinic, vicarious liability of the radiologist is of no consequence since the employing health care facility would be legally responsible for negligent acts committed by either of them. In private offices owned and operated by radiologists, the radiologist-employer would be vicariously liable for any negligence of the technologist-employee.[7]

Liability for Acts of Residents

Although the hospital or university that employs radiology residents generally assumes primary liability for their negligent actions, attending radiologists may nevertheless be forced to vicariously share this liability, either through the borrowed servant doctrine (as described above) or the tort of *negligent supervision*.[8] Indeed, one appellate court ruled an attending physician was liable for malpractice even though the resident had been found innocent, arguing that an attending physician should be held to a higher standard of care than a resident.[9]

Various courts in nonradiology contexts have attempted to define "adequate supervision" as it relates to attending physicians and residents. The general concept is that radiologists must use their own best judgment to determine how much supervision is necessary, based on an assessment of the competency level of the resident and the overriding need to ensure optimum patient care in appropriately interpreting imaging examinations and performing radiologic procedures. Courts have stressed that faculty members at a medical center "serve dual purposes; they teach and they care for patients.... As long as the faculty physician undertakes to care for a patient (whether directly administering the care or delegating that responsibility to others," they will not be immunized from liability.[10] With relation to a surgical (and, by extension, radiologic) procedure, one court[11] has observed that even though it "was actually performed by a resident, defendants were under a duty to see that it was performed properly. It is their skill and training as specialists which enables them to judge the competency of the resident's performance." Consequently, the court rejected the claim that supervision of a patient's care "does not constitute the practice of medicine," stressing that the liability of the faculty surgeons "was not predicated on the negligence of the resident, but upon their own negligence in failing to provide adequate supervision." Faculty physicians can be liable for negligent supervision even when they are not actually present. As one court stated in response to an obstetrician's claim that he did not have a duty to personally examine each patient while he was on call or to intervene in the treatment of a patient unless asked to do so by a resident or other hospital personnel, "Simply remaining at home and available to take telephone calls is not always an acceptable standard of care for supervision of residents."[12]

The federal government has attempted to define the supervisory relationship between residents and attending physicians by amending the rules for Medicare reimbursement. Initially, teaching physicians were entitled to bill Medicare in their own names for medical services that were actually rendered by residents whom they supervised. After audits revealed that the level of such supervision was often extremely low, new policies were instituted. All radiographic examinations must be performed under at least a "general" level of attending physician supervision; some require either "direct" or "personal" supervision. These terms have been defined as follows[13]:

General supervision: the radiologist's presence is not required during performance of the procedure (plain radiographs of the extremities, pelvis, spine, skull, chest, and abdomen; ultrasound).
Direct supervision: the radiologist is not required to be in the room during the procedure, but must be in the area and immediately available to provide assistance (CT, MRI, nuclear medicine, and radiologic examinations using contrast material).
Personal supervision: the radiologist must be present in the room during performance of the procedure (interventional procedures).

These Medicare rules have increased the level of faculty supervision of residents, as has the move in some hospitals to provide 24-hour radiologic coverage by attending radiologists.[14,15]

Liability of Chairpersons Administering Departments

Chairpersons of radiology departments have been named as defendants in malpractice lawsuits for alleged acts of negligence arising from their roles as department administrators. Charges of misconduct may include allegations of failure to (a) develop or implement department policies designed to ensure good patient care; (b) supervise department personnel, residents, or associate radiologists; or (c) provide efficient and timely reporting of radiologic examinations.[16] Courts have distinguished between chairpersons directly charged with supervision of residents in the care of patients (where they would be no different from other attending physicians) and those performing administrative duties in their role of chair or program director.[17] In the latter category, some have found chairpersons liable for "failing to provide medically acceptable rules and regulations which would ensure appropriate supervision of all patients."[18] Other disagree, maintaining that although a departmental chairperson may be "ultimately responsible" for all patients in the department, this cannot mean that the chairperson "undertook an obligation of treat every patient in the medical center" requiring the services of the department.[19]

The liability of a department chairperson also may depend on the type of practice. The concept of *governmental immunity* provides that municipal or state officials who are performing the duties of their statutory offices with good faith and judgment are not liable personally for damages relating to injuries resulting from their official acts. Thus various officials in state university or public hospitals, including program directors and department chairs, are protected from liability incurred during performance of their administrative duties.[20] Therefore, there is a greater likelihood that a chairperson in a private hospital will be held liable for "administrative malpractice" than one in a state- or municipally-owned hospital.[21]

Liability for Acts of Partners

Partners are legally considered agents of each other. Therefore, they are liable for professional negligence committed by other partners in carrying out activities related to the business of the partnership, "even if they do not participate in, ratify or have knowledge of such torts."

Hospital Liability for Acts of Physicians

As charitable institutions, hospitals historically were granted absolute immunity from tort liability and any application of the doctrine of *respondeat superior*. This was based on the concept that since the hospital was unable to control the members of its staff (physicians, nurses, and other skilled professionals) or dictate the treatment they provide, it could not be held liable for its employees' negligence.[23] A court decision in 1914 held that a hospital could be vicariously liability for the "administrative" acts of its employees, but not for negligent conduct related to the medical care of patients.[24] Hospital immunity was over-turned almost a half century later,[25] though vicarious liability was initially limited to negligent acts committed by physicians and nurses *employed* by the hospital and not for the actions of nonemployed medical staff or hospital-based physicians who were considered *independent contractors*. During the past 20 years, however, there is a growing trend for courts to impose vicarious liability on hospitals for the negligent acts of independent-contractor physicians.[26] For example, a federal district court found a hospital liable for an independent-contractor radiologist's negligence in not promptly communicating the results of an imaging study to the referring physician.[27] The court ruled that prompt reporting was an administrative responsibility and that the physician was functioning as an agent of the hospital when relaying the report. In another case,[28] a court found a hospital to be the employer of a nonsalaried radiologist based on the hospital's legal right to control the professional performance of medical staff members, the exclusiveness of the contract, the hospital's role as billing agent, and the patient's lack of choice in selecting a radiologist. The court declined to be bound by a statement in the hospital admission form, signed by the patient, acknowledging that the radiologist was an independent contractor and not a hospital employee.[29]

In many states, there has been a shift in judicial focus from examining the details of the hospital-physician relationship to an assessment of how the relationship would appear to the reasonable patient. Courts increasingly have held that health care facilities encourage the public to believe that hospital-based physicians (radiologists, pathologists, anesthesiologists, and emergency room physicians) are hospital employees or agents, even if they are technically independent contractors. Rather than assess the traditional criterion of the degree of control exerted by the employer (the hospital) over the employee/independent contractor (the physician), courts have developed a two-factor test to determine if a hospital is vicariously liable for negligent acts committed by its physicians: (a) whether the patient looks to the hospital, rather than to the individual physician, for medical care; and (b) whether the hospital holds out that the physician is its employee.[30] In most instances, patients select a specific hospital for their overall health care based on its prestige, location, or special programs, and then as a matter of course have their diagnostic studies performed in the imaging department of that facility. Therefore, even though a radiologist may technically be an independent contractor, most patients consider them as hospital employees. This "apparent agency" is sufficient for courts to treat these radiologists as if they were employees, thus making the hospital vicariously liability for any of their negligent acts.[31]

The expansion of vicarious liability of hospitals for the negligent acts of independent-contractor physicians may have significant ramifications on radiologists who work and bill separately from the hospitals in which they practice. Hospitals forced to assume increasing legal responsibility for radiologists within their facilities may attempt to exert tighter control on the manner in which they practice, taking a more active role in ensuring the quality of imaging services rather than delegating this to their independent-contractor radiologists. In many instances, this may be effectively the same as the requirements imposed for years by the Joint Commission on Accreditation of Health Organizations (but conveniently ignored by hospital management).[32]

Hospital-based, nonsalaried radiologists who bill independently can take steps to decrease the chance of being considered employees of the hospitals in which they practice. Signs placed in strategic locations throughout the radiology department can indicate that the radiologists are in private fee-for-service practice, and similar information can be included on billing forms. When questioned by physician colleagues, hospital employees, or patients, such radiologists should clearly state that they are not hospital employees.[33]

Hospitals also can be liable for the consequences of breaches of duties owed directly to the patient. These include maintenance of buildings and grounds; selection and maintenance of equipment; proper selection and supervision of employees; proper selection and monitoring of medical staff; and providing adequate security.[34]

Endnotes

1 *Baker v. Story*, 621 SW2d 639 (Tex App 1981).
2 Miller RD, Hutton RC. *Problems in Health Care Law, 8th ed.* Gaithersburg (MD), Aspen, 2000, pg. 380.
3 *Petrovich v Share Health Plan*, Lexis 148 (Ill App 1998).
4 Berlin L. Liability of radiologists when supervising technologists. *AJR* 1999;172:285–289.
5 Ibid.
6 Ibid.
7 Ibid.
8 Berlin L. Liability of attending physicians when supervising residents. *AJR* 1998;171:295–298.
9 *Baker v. Story*, 621 SW2d 639 (Tex App 1981).
10 *Klein v Boyle et al*, 776 F Supp 285 (West. Dis. VA 1991).
11 *McCullough v Hutzel Hospital*, 276 NW2d 569 (Mich App 1979).

12 *Rouse v Pitt County Memorial Hospital et al*, 470 SE2d 44 (NC 1996).
13 Berlin L. Liability of attending physicians when supervising residents. *AJR* 1998;171:295–298.
14 Spigos D, Freedy L, Mueller C. 24-hour coverage by attending physicians: a new paradigm. *AJR* 1996;167:1089–1090.
15 Steele RD, Kerr HH. 24-hour radiology. *AJR* 1997;169:953–954.
16 Berlin L. Liability of chairpersons when administering radiology departments. *AJR* 2000;175:967-972.
17 Ibid.
18 *Maxwell v Cole*, 482 NYS2d 1000 (NY 1984).
19 *Klein v Boyle et al*, 776 F Supp 285 (West. Dis. VA 1991).
20 Reuter SR. Professional liability in postgraduate medical education: who is liable for resident negligence? *J Leg Med* 1994;15:485-531.
21 Berlin L. Liability of chairpersons when administering radiology departments. *AJR* 2000;175:967-972.
22 *Schmitz v St. Lukes Hospital et al* (D.N.D. 1966).
23 Boumil MM, Elias CE. *The Law of Medical Liability*. St. Paul, MN: West Publishing, 1995.
24 *Schloendorff v Society of New York Hospital*, 105 NE 92 (NY 1914).
25 *Bing v Thunig*, 143 NE2d 3 (NY 1957).
26 Berlin L. Vicarious liability. *AJR* 1997;169:621-624.
27 *Keene v Methodist Hospital* 324 F. Suppl 231 (N.D. Ind. 1971).
28 *Beeck v Tucson General Hospital* 18 Ariz App. 165, 500 P.2d 1153 (1972).
29 Miller RD, Hutton RC. *Problems in Health Care Law, 8th ed*. Gaithersburg (MD), Aspen, 2000, pg. 318.
30 *Jackson v Power*, 743 P2d 1376 (Alaska 1987).
31 *Marek v Professional Health Services*, 432 A.2d 538 (NJ 1981).
32 Berlin L. Vicarious liability. *AJR* 1997;169:621-624.
33 Ibid.
34 Miller RD, Hutton RC. *Problems in Health Care Law, 8th ed*. Gaithersburg (MD), Aspen, 2000, pgs. 382-388.

3
Standards and Practice Guidelines

A growing trend within the medical community is the establishment of written standards and practice guidelines. Developed by groups of national experts, they can be used in malpractice litigation to replace the traditional notion of "community standards," which need to be interpreted by one or more expert witnesses at trial. Guidelines pertaining to radiology have also been issued by Congress and regulatory agencies, such as the rules and regulations developed by the Food and Drug Administration mandating practices at mammography facilities as part of the Mammography Quality Standards Act (MQSA) of 1992.[1] Because these guidelines can be used as evidence of appropriate medical practice, whether the physician complied with the guidelines may be relevant to an issue that is basic to every malpractice case: Did the conduct of the defendant fall within the appropriate standard of care?

Without any standards, recommendations, or guidelines issued by a medical specialty society, a defendant is effectively held to a standard of care that reflects the bias of the plaintiff's expert witness. This has resulted in increasing damage awards, inconsistent verdicts, and excessive reliance on expert testimony. Verdicts are often based on a jury's inadequate understanding of medical facts, causation, and the duty of care. They are often influenced by such intangibles as the courtroom charisma of the attorneys and expert witnesses or the relative attractiveness of the plaintiff or the defendant. The goal of practice standards is to increase the fairness of professional liability litigation by providing judges and juries with clear, informative guidelines for evaluating evidence. It is hoped that this goal will reduce the random nature of the professional liability system by providing a more predictable and fairer way to assess medical outcomes.[2] In addition to eliminating the "battle of the experts," practice standards could reduce litigation costs and even lead to lower insurance premiums, since attorney fees, along with the cost of administering liability insurance, account for at least two thirds of each dollar paid for malpractice professional liability insurance.[3]

Standards and practice guidelines have been admitted into evidence both by plaintiffs as "inculpatory" (tending to prove blameworthiness) evidence of the defendant's violation of the standard of care, and by defendants as "exculpatory" (tending to prove innocence) evidence that the standard of care was met. Plaintiffs may argue that noncompliance with an established standard automatically establishes negligence ("negligence per se"), though the courts have not extended this theory to standards developed in other industries and thus would probably not apply it to guidelines established by medical societies. Conversely, defendants may claim that adherence to a standard necessarily means that they were not negligent. However, this theory also would probably be unsuccessful because courts generally view compliance with a law as the *minimum* level of acceptable behavior and not necessarily one that reflects the prevailing standard of care.[4]

Standards and guidelines generally are considered admissible as evidence, though courts exercise discretion as to the weight they should be given. Indeed, a court may reach conclusions contrary to the practice guidelines if it finds that other evidence about the standard is more persuasive. One court refused to admit into evidence a pamphlet titled "Standards for Ambulatory Care," stating that the contents appeared to be recommendations rather than standards. Conversely, despite arguments by another defendant that the guidelines of the American Society of Anesthesiologists relied on by the plaintiff were only "emerging" and were not "mandatory" but rather "encouraged," the court held that such guidelines "necessarily embody what a reasonably prudent [physician] would do" and thus constituted evidence of the standard of care.[5]

Risk management guidelines promulgated by private insurance carriers do not carry the same legal weight as those issued by established governmental agencies or professional societies.[6] As one court observed: "The express purpose of the risk management guidelines was to attempt to 'decrease the possibility of a malpractice case, increase the possibility of prevailing or decrease the eventual loss,'" and as such it "did not reflect a generally recognized standard of care within the medical profession."[7]

At times, courts are faced with guidelines of two societies that disagree. In such cases, the court generally employs the so-called *two schools of thought doctrine*, which permits the physician to be found not negligent for following a minority approach "so long as it is reputable and respected by reasonable medical experts."[8]

What is the effect of an absence of guidelines? In one case, the absence of a recommendation by the American Cancer Society to perform prostate-specific antigen tests for detecting prostate cancer did not exculpate the defendant physician who failed to order it. However, as more guidelines are developed, defenses based on the absence of a specific guideline may become more successful, and the absence of a recommendation may carry greater weight.

American College of Radiology Standards

The American College of Radiology (ACR), the preeminent professional society of radiologists, has promulgated a long list of standards dealing with all aspects of diagnostic imaging and interventional procedures.[9] These written guidelines exert substantial influence on what the medical and legal communities perceive to be the radiology standard of care. Despite the fact that the ACR precedes each written standard with a disclaimer stating that the standards are "not rules" but rather "defined principles of practice which should generally produce high quality radiologic care," the standards are considered by many professionals and lay people as mandatory regulations. Radiologists should be aware that the standards of practice are continually being revised, reflecting the rapid changes in scientific knowledge and the development of more sophisticated imaging techniques.[10]

Departmental Standards[11]

All radiology facilities are required to establish written policies and procedures that govern the conduct of their practice. These include (but are not limited to) the techniques and projections for various imaging examinations, clinical indications for specific studies, and procedures to be followed for communicating results to referring physicians and patients. Individual radiologists should carefully follow these policies and review them on a regular basis. Any policy that is impractical or difficult to follow should be modified so that full compliance is possible. When writing or referring to departmental policies, it is essential to pay close attention to the verbs used. Words such as "may" or "recommend" suggest some flexibility in the implementation of the policy; in contrast, "should" permits less flexibility and "must" or "shall/will be" preclude any variation from the written standard.

At times, radiologists may be convinced that proper patient care in a specific case requires deviation from the written protocols. In such a situation, it is essential that the radiologist document the reason for the variation in the radiology report, a note in the patient's chart, or a log kept in the radiology department.

Legal Effect of Standards and Practice Guidelines

In addition to improving patient care, standards and practice guidelines initially were established to diminish the incidence of malpractice litigation and related costs.[12] Theoretically, if radiologists strictly follow standards and practice guidelines, the quality of care will improve, fewer injuries will occur, and less malpractice claims will be filed. The number of spurious claims may be reduced if more explicit guidelines about what constitutes appropriate care can help attorneys better assess whether negligence has occurred and the case is likely to succeed. A commonly accepted, more precisely defined standard of care ideally would make legal proceedings shorter and less costly. Rather than being encumbered by the need to establish the standard of care, the legal process could focus on whether extenuating circumstances mitigated the application of the standard in the particular case. Conversely, however, one could argue that the promulgation of standards and practice guidelines could increase the number of malpractice claims. Studies have shown that there are five to eight times more injuries resulting from negligence than there are claims filed. Thus, if guidelines serve to define malpractice more precisely, attorneys may be able to identify some meritorious cases that are not currently pursued.

Despite optimistic projections of the positive effects of standards to protect physicians, the results have not been encouraging. In a report on practice guidelines and malpractice litigation issued in 1994,[13] researchers at the Harvard School of Public Health found that the guidelines were used three times more often against physicians (to inculpate) than in their defense (to exculpate), and that plaintiffs were successful in almost 75% of cases in which guidelines were cited at trial. Instead of reducing costs by decreasing the need for expert witnesses, just the opposite effect occurred. In the same year, a newspaper article[14] termed practice guidelines "powerful weapons for plaintiffs in malpractice cases," and a lawyer gleefully observed that he and other plaintiffs' attorneys are using them in court to show that physicians are not following the minimum standards of care detailed by their own professional organizations.

State Legislation[15]

The anticipated cost savings related to the widespread use of practice standards primarily depends on their eliminating the need for expert witnesses. This requires action by the state legislatures recognizing these guidelines as defining the appropriate standard of care. To accomplish this task, state officials and representatives from the medical, legal, and lay communities must approve, adopt, and announce the guidelines that would govern medical practice. Several state legislatures have already enacted legislation permitting standards to be used as an "affirmative defense," allowing physician-defendants who follow designated protocols to be found not liable for malpractice. However, at this time plaintiffs cannot use the guidelines to inculpate physicians who do no adhere to them.

Even if promulgated standards are given the force of law, it is important for radiologists and other physicians to remember that the duty they owe to their patients overrides the duty to blindly follow such guidelines. In some cases, it will be essential that physicians seek exemptions from the legally mandated standards in order to provide their patients with optimal care.

Endnotes

1 Berlin L. Standard of care. *AJR* 1998;170:275-278.
2 *Medical-Legal Issues for Residents in Radiology.* Reston, VA: American College of Radiology, 1994:51.
3 Tzeel A. Clinical practice guidelines and medical malpractice. *The Physician Executive*, March-April 2002:36-39.
4 *Medical-Legal Issues for Residents in Radiology.* Reston, VA: American College of Radiology 1994:50.
5 *Washington v Washington Hospital Center*, 579 A2d 177 (DC App 1990).
6 Berlin L. Standard of care. *AJR* 1998;170:275-278.
7 *Quigley v Jobe*, 851 P2d 236 (Colo App 1992).
8 *Levine v Rosen*, 616 A2d 623 (PA 1992).
9 *ACR Standards 2000-2001.* Reston, VA: American College of Radiology, 2000.
10 Berlin L. Standard of care. *AJR* 1998;170:275-278.
11 Ibid.
12 Ibid.
13 Hyams AL, Brandenburg JA, Lipsitz, Brennan TA. *Report to Physician Payment Review Commission: Practice Guidelines and Malpractice Litigation.* Boston: Harvard School of Public Health, Department of Health Policy and Management, 1994.

14 Felsenthal E. Doctors' own guidelines hurt them in court. *Wall Street Journal* October 19, 1994:B1,B12.

15 Tzeel A. Clinical practice guidelines and medical malpractice. *The Physician Executive*, March-April 2002:36-39.

4
Anatomy of a Malpractice Lawsuit

Malpractice lawsuits are civil actions that are almost always filed in state courts. Consequently, the specific procedures that must be followed are governed by the rules and regulations of that particular state. Most patients who believe that they have been harmed (suffered damages) by the negligent conduct of a physician consult an attorney to represent them. Although any person can file a lawsuit, almost all prefer to be represented by an attorney who is familiar with the often-complicated formal legal procedures and rules of law of the state.

Unlike most civil cases, in which an attorney is remunerated at a stipulated per hour rate for the time spent, attorneys handling malpractice lawsuits usually work on the basis of a *contingency fee*—a percentage of any financial award eventually granted to the plaintiff. This contingency fee typically varies from 25% to 33% of the final judgment award or settlement, subject to specific state-imposed restrictions (especially for "pain and suffering" of the plaintiff). Because malpractice attorneys must invest large amounts of time in what typically is a lengthy process that may last 5 years or more, they must carefully evaluate the merits of the case before agreeing to represent a client. This evaluation frequently entails consultations with physician experts to determine the validity of the plaintiff's claim and the likelihood of its success. The existence of a contingency fee system results in many meritorious suits never being filed; even if the negligence of a physician is clear, a malpractice attorney will not agree to handle a case in which the damages are relatively slight so that any monetary award (and the percentage received by the lawyer) would not even cover expenses.

Prefiling Procedures

Many states prescribe specific procedures that must be satisfied before a lawsuit may be filed. Some mandate the convening of a screening medical panel to provide a preliminary evaluation of the case. This panel, which may be composed exclusively of physicians or also include attorneys and laypersons, hears the plaintiff's case and may issue a nonbinding opinion. Even if the assessment is not favorable, the plaintiff can still bring the case to court. However, some states allow the panel's findings to be introduced as evidence in any subsequent adjudication. Some states require the plaintiff to provide a notice of intent to sue. Both of these procedures are designed to offer a way to informally resolve potential conflicts and avoid formal legal proceedings.

Formal Filing

As with any civil action, the plaintiff begins a malpractice lawsuit by a filing in the appropriate court a *complaint* that specifies the judicial relief sought against specified defendants. In addition to giving notice, this initial action is also intended to narrow and formulate the issues involved in the case so that all parties can make appropriate pretrial and trial preparation. Although some states (including California, Illinois, and New York) have highly technical requirements, most states have adopted the more liberal federal rules. The complaint must contain a "short and plain statement of the [basic facts of the] claim showing that the pleader is entitled to relief."[1] This and all other papers filed with the court require the signature of the attorney (or the party, if not represented), certifying that after "reasonable inquiry" the filing is (a) well-grounded in fact; (b) warranted by existing law or a good-faith argument for the extension, modification, or reversal of existing law; and (c) not introduced for any improper purpose such as delay or harassment.[2] This rule is designed to deter lawyers for plaintiffs from asserting claims that have no basis in law or fact, as well as to prevent them from bringing in peripheral defendants with minimal connection to the case. The filing of frivolous claims can lead to sanctions, most commonly the awarding of attorneys' fees to the opposing party. Once an action is commenced by the filing of a complaint, the plaintiff has 120 days to serve the complaint on the defendant.[3]

A physician receiving notice of intent to sue or a formal legal complaint must immediately notify his or her professional liability carrier, which will assign an attorney to the case. This attorney will review the complaint, contact the physician, and discuss the proper approach to the situation. The physician should feel free to discuss all aspects of the case freely with the attorney, since all such communications are protected by attorney-client privilege. Within a specified period that varies among jurisdictions, the defense issues an *answer*, in which it must admit, deny, or plead lack of knowledge sufficient to respond to the allegations in the complaint.[4] A denial must be made in good faith after a reasonable inquiry into the facts at issue. Although the defense may issue a *general* denial that denies each and every material allegation of the complaint, it is far more common to offer a *specific* denial aimed at certain allegations. For example, the defendant may deny negligence, while admitting that an injury occurred. There must be a response to each allegation in the complaint; those allegations (other than the amount of damages) that are not explicitly denied are deemed admitted.[5] The answer also must explicitly assert any applicable *affirmative defenses*[6] —claims that seek to avoid the legal effect of the opposing party's allegations without actually denying them. In effect, affirmative defenses argue that the defendant should not be found liable even assuming the alleged facts to be true. Designed to prevent the plaintiff from being surprised by the defense at trial, these affirmative defenses include contributory negligence on the part of the plaintiff (see page 17) and the statute of limitations (see page 15).

It may be possible to file a motion to dismiss, asserting that the plaintiff improperly filed the lawsuit or drafted the complaint. Among the most cited technical deficiencies are the inability of the plaintiff to state a sufficient cause of action, failure to bring the suit within the statute of limitations, and failure to adhere to local rules. For example, in Illinois the complaint in a medical malpractice lawsuit must be accompanied by an expert affidavit, in which a health care provider who has analyzed the medical record asserts that there is a meritorious case against the defendant. A motion to dismiss may be "with prejudice," meaning that the action cannot be refiled, or merely "without prejudice" (dismissal for technical reasons with the plaintiff allowed the opportunity to refile).[7]

Discovery

Discovery is the term applied to the pretrial activities in the litigation process to determine the essential questions and issues in dispute, as well as the evidence that each party plans to present at trial so that neither side can unfairly surprise the other. Discovery can help eliminate fictitious issues, claims, or defenses by revealing overwhelming evidence on one side, thereby paving the way for a settlement or summary disposition. In general, parties "may obtain discovery regarding any matter not privileged, which is relevant to the subject matter in the pending action."[8] The information sought does not necessarily have to be admissible as proof in court; all that is required is that it be "reasonably calculated to lead to the discovery of admissible evidence." The defendant's general financial resources usually have no bearing on the issues to be presented at trial and thus are irrelevant for purposes of discovery. Nevertheless, the existence and extent of any insurance coverage is discoverable (even though insurance is not relevant to any issue in the case) because of the belief that knowledge of the insurance might foster settlement.[9]

To enable all parties to present a full case, each party may require the other to provide a written and signed statement (a) identifying each person whom the other party expects to call as an expert witness at trial; (b) stating the subject matter on which the expert is expected to testify; and (c) stating the substance of the facts and opinions to which the expert is expected to testify and a summary of the ground for each opinion.[10] However, immunity from discovery is given to the opinions of experts that counsel has consulted in *preparation* of the case but is not planning to actually call to testify at trial.[11]

There are several methods to secure disclosure of information during the discovery process. In malpractice lawsuits, the plaintiff always requests the defense to provide relevant medical records and imaging studies. *Interrogatories* are a set of formal printed questions submitted to an opposing party to be answered before and in preparation for trial.[12] The written answers to these questions, which are prepared within 30 days with the assistance of an attorney, must be signed and affirmed as true. The major disadvantage of interrogatories is that they afford the discovering party little flexibility, since there is no opportunity to rephrase or follow up a question based on the response of the opposing party. Therefore, by far the most important discovery procedure is the oral deposition.[13]

Deposition

A deposition is an oral examination by the opposing counsel of a witness under oath that takes place out of court but in a trial-like setting in the presence of a court reporter, who prepares an accurate transcript of the testimony and any objections raised. In a malpractice lawsuit, depositions are used to obtain testimony from both the plaintiff and defendant(s), as well as expert witnesses who are to testify at any upcoming trial. Prior to the proceeding, the person to be deposed typically reviews anticipated questions with the attorney representing the party or calling the witness. The rules governing the questions that may be asked during a deposition are not as strict as the rules of evidence in court, since the procedure is primarily designed to help each party assess the position of the other. Objections asserted are noted on the record and may be renewed at trial in an effort to keep the answers from the jury, but the witness must answer the questions posed by opposing counsel. All statements made at a deposition (as well as interrogatories) are preserved and may be either introduced into evidence at trial if it is impossible for a witness to attend in person, or used during cross-examination to impeach contradictory testimony at trial.

Because attorneys in malpractice suits often wish to secure the services of well-known experts in various locations across the country, video depositions have become increasingly common. Video depositions substantially decrease travel expenses and are more effective than transcribed testimony if a witness will not be available at trial.

Settlement Attempts

Following discovery, attempts at settlement are usually made to avoid the expenditure of extensive resources required for a court trial. In some states, mandatory pretrial settlement conferences are required by law (see below). If a settlement is reached, formal legal documents are prepared for the parties to sign. This final disposition of the case has the same impact against reassertion of future claims regarding the same matter as the verdict at a trial. The legal principle of *res judicata*, which is similar to its criminal-law counterpart of "double jeopardy," prevents a retrial of issues that have been *legally settled* by mutual agreement or a judicial proceeding.[14]

There are many factors to consider in deciding whether to settle or take a case to trial. "The most important factor is the careful and impartial analysis of the medical issues, and the opportunity to prevail at trial." The insurance company generally views the issue as a pure business decision, while the radiologist must weigh the fact that any settlement (or adverse jury finding) will be reported to the National Data Bank, may lead to investigation by the state licensing committee, and results in increased rates for professional liability insurance.[15]

Pretrial Conference

Many states, and the federal system, give the judge authority to conduct a *pretrial conference* to (a) simplify or clarify the issues in the case; (b) obtain stipulations and admissions of fact to streamline the proceedings; (c) identify witnesses to be presented at trial; and (d) facilitate handling of the case through scheduling and judicial management. A key function of the pretrial conference is to promote settlement. Although the court is not authorized to dictate the terms of a settlement, it may suggest guidelines for the parties to follow. Some judges, anxious to clear their dockets, use "persuasion" that verges on coercion in trying to bring about a settlement; however, judges who go too far in trying to get the parties to settle may find themselves reversed on appeal.

Summary Judgment

Summary judgment is a method for avoiding the unnecessary delay and expense of a trial if one party can demonstrate that the evidentiary material shows that there is "no genuine issue of material fact" and that he or she is "entitled to judgment as a matter of law."[16] This determination, made by the judge and based on pretrial written submissions and deposition transcripts, essentially requires that "no reasonable jury could find for the opposing party." Summary judgment must be distinguished from a directed verdict and a judgment notwithstanding the verdict, both of which depend on trial testimony (see below).

In most cases, the defendant moves for summary judgment by claiming that the plaintiff has failed to come forward with sufficient evidence to support a verdict in the plantiff's favor. Because the plaintiff bears the burden of proof at trial, the defense does not necessarily have to provide any depositions or other supporting evidentiary materials. Instead, the defense may be entitled to summary judgment merely by showing that the existing record contains no evidence that would allow the plaintiff to prove an essential element of its case. The plaintiff can move for summary judgment by arguing that the evidence is so strong that a reasonable jury could only find for him or her. Regardless of which party moves for summary judgment, all the evidence must be construed most favorably to the party *opposing* the motion, even if it is highly unlikely that the opposing party would be likely to prevail at trial. Denial of summary judgment is not immediately appealable to a higher court. However, a grant of summary judgment may be immediately appealed to a higher court if it results in a final judgment. On review, the appellate court has plenary power and does not have to give deference to the trial judge's decision.

Trial

Malpractice lawsuits are usually tried before a jury, though the parties can waive a jury trial and have the judge serve as both the finder of fact and the decider of law. A jury is selected from a representative panel of citizens in a procedure (*voir dire*) in which the counsels for both sides ask each prospective juror questions designed to discover whether he or she is biased or has a connection with a party in the case or any prospective witness.[17] A juror who demonstrates such bias or reports a connection can be dismissed *for cause*; there is no limit to the number of challenges that may be made to eliminate jurors for these reasons since they are predicated on the need to find an impartial jury. Each party is also entitled to a limited number of *peremptory challenges* (generally no more than six)—the right to dismiss a juror without having to specify any reason ("*without cause*").

Once a jury has been seated, the attorney for the plaintiff (who bears the burden of proof) presents an opening statement. The defense attorney then is given the choice of making an opening statement or deferring it until later in the trial when the defense presents its case. The plaintiff then calls its witnesses to present direct evidence, with cross-examination by the defendant; subsequently, the roles are reversed. In a jury trial, either party may move for a *directed verdict* at the close of evidence offered by the adversary. In essence, the moving party is arguing that the evidence demonstrates that he or she must prevail and thus there is no reason to send the case to the jury.[18] For example, the defendant may move for a directed verdict by arguing that the plaintiff has failed to prove a necessary element of the cause of action (such as the existence of a duty or causation in a malpractice suit based on the theory of negligence).

If the motion for a directed verdict is denied, both sides may offer rebuttal evidence and then present their closing arguments, with the plaintiff getting the first and last of the three arguments. The judge then instructs the jury as to the relevant law (not the factual merits). Generally, the instructions are drafted by the parties and approved by the court. The jury then retires to discuss the case until it reaches a verdict, which is based on the standard of *preponderance of the evidence*—more likely than not (or 51% likely on a scale of 100%) that the physician's conduct resulted in the patient's injury. In federal and most state courts, the verdict must be unanimous unless the parties agree otherwise.[19] However, some states permit non-unanimous verdicts, as does California, where in civil cases only three fourths of the jury must concur.[20]

Even after it is rendered, a jury verdict may be nullified by the judge. Known as *judgment notwithstanding the verdict* (in Latin, judgment *non obstante veredicto* (JNOV)), it can be granted if the judge determines that the jury verdict based on the evidence was unreasonable as a matter of law. The judge also has wide discretion to grant a motion for a new trial based on any miscarriage of justice. Unlike a directed verdict or JNOV, such a ruling does not end the case or infringe on the right to a jury trial. The most common grounds for granting a new trial are (a) errors of law at trial (e.g., an erroneous instruction regarding the burden of proof); (b) a verdict contrary to the manifest weight of the evidence; (c) improper or irregular conduct ("prejudicial misconduct") at the trial by the judge, the attorneys, or the jury; (d) the discovery of significant new evidence; and (e) a verdict that was clearly or grossly inadequate or excessive.[21]

Appeal

The losing party may file an appeal to obtain review by a higher court. This normally does not involve a retrial of the factual material in the case or the introduction of new evidence, but rather is limited to a consideration of the rulings by the trial court in light of the record on which those rulings were made. Sources of an appeal may include alleged errors concerning the admission or exclusion of evidence or the language of jury instructions. Counsel must have properly preserved the right to appeal by making a timely objection, and the appealing party is limited to arguments made in the trial court.

Appellate courts are extremely deferential to jury verdicts and their underlying factual findings. Discretionary rulings by the trial judge, such as orders on procedural or evidentiary matters, may be reversed only if there has been a clear abuse of discretion or failure to apply the correct legal standards. The appellate court cannot simply reverse a trial court judgment because it does not agree with the result. Rather, there must have been a *prejudicial error*, i.e., one that affected the substantial rights of the party and was not merely "harmless" error.[22]

Endnotes

1 Federal Rules of Civil Procedure, Rule 8(a).
2 Federal Rules of Civil Procedure, Rule 11.
3 Federal Rules of Civil Procedure, Rule 3.
4 Federal Rules of Civil Procedure, Rule 8(b).
5 Federal Rules of Civil Procedure, Rule 8(d).
6 Federal Rules of Civil Procedure, Rule 8(c).
7 Petrek RF Jr, Slovis MR. The defendant in a malpractice suit: an integral part of the defense team. *Pediatr Radiol* 1998;28:905–912.
8 Federal Rules of Civil Procedure, Rule 26(b).
9 Federal Rules of Civil Procedure, Rule 26(b)(2).
10 Federal Rules of Civil Procedure, Rule 26(b)(4).
11 Ibid.

12 Federal Rules of Civil Procedure, Rule 33.

13 Federal Rules of Civil Procedure, Rule 30.

14 Brenner RJ. Breast imaging: screening and diagnostic mammography. In: *Risk Management: Test and Syllabus*. Reston, VA: American College of Radiology, 1999:1–7.

15 Petrek RF Jr, Slovis MR. The defendant in a malpractice suit: an integral part of the defense team. *Pediatr Radiol* 1998;28:905–912.

16 Federal Rules of Civil Procedure, Rule 56.

17 Federal Rules of Civil Procedure, Rule 47(a).

18 Federal Rules of Civil Procedure, Rule 50(a).

19 Federal Rules of Civil Procedure, Rule 48.

20 California Civil Procedures Code §618.

21 Federal Rules of Civil Procedure, Rule 59.

22 Federal Rules of Civil Procedure, Rule 61.

5
Expert Witnesses

Availability

In malpractice litigation, the testimony of expert witnesses is essential to establish the applicable standard of medical care and whether or not the defendant deviated from it. The plaintiff, who bears the initial burden of proof, usually must offer the testimony of an expert witness or risk a directed verdict for the defendant. In the past, securing expert testimony was often a difficult task for a plaintiff, primarily due to a "conspiracy of silence" among physicians, especially in small rural locations, who felt that it was morally objectionable, perhaps disloyal, to testify against "one's own." There was a well-founded fear of retaliation by colleagues if the expert later became a defendant, as well as the concern that physicians who became involved in legal matters might not get future referrals from other doctors in the community. The unavailability of experts willing to testify for the plaintiff led to the emergence of "hired guns"—physicians who made a practice of becoming involved in litigation and often were willing to attest to anything that would bolster the plaintiff's case. These generally unscrupulous individuals attempted to testify in a wide variety of cases, regardless of whether they possessed any genuine expertise in a particular field. This led to the adoption of increasingly strict qualifications for expert witnesses.[1]

In addition to limited availability, plaintiffs may have difficulty securing expert witnesses because of the expense involved. Physicians often charge high fees (sometimes unconscionable) to serve as an expert witness. To render an opinion, the expert must acquire substantial familiarity with the plaintiff's case and issue a report before trial, which may involve numerous billable hours and substantial costs. If the case is being handled on a contingency basis, the cost of expert witnesses must be paid up front by the plaintiff's attorney, regardless of whether there is a favorable outcome. Consequently, many meritorious cases are never pursued, primarily because of the prohibitive cost of expert witnesses.[2]

In contrast to the difficulties experienced by malpractice plaintiffs in finding expert witnesses, defendants are generally much more successful in finding colleagues willing to support their positions. Nevertheless, many physicians prefer not to get involved on either side, due to the time commitment, the need to be available for trial at unpredictable times, and an overall dislike of the litigation process. Today, many courts have addressed the burdensome nature of the legal process by permitting videotaped expert testimony, obviating the need for an expert witness to actually testify at trial.[3]

The American College of Radiology (ACR) has recognized that fair and just adjudication of cases of alleged radiologist malpractice obligates members of the specialty to serve as expert witnesses and testify in court when appropriate.[4] Similarly, the American Medical Association states that physicians, as citizens and as professionals with special training and experience, have an ethical obligation to serve as expert witnesses to improve the administration of justice.[5]

Role

Expert witnesses possess special knowledge, skill, experience, training, or education that permits them to testify to an opinion that can aid the judge and jury in resolving a question that is beyond the understanding or competence of laypersons.[6] Under common law, unless the expert's opinion was based on first-hand observation (as in the case of a treating physicians testifying about the diagnoses of their patients), the facts on which the opinion was based generally had to be admitted into evidence to establish a foundation. The Federal Rules of Evidence have relaxed this requirement and permit the expert to rely on inadmissible facts or data, as long as it is "of a type reasonably relied upon by experts in the particular field in forming opinions or inferences upon the subject."[7] Thus in addition to first-hand observation, the expert can rely on statements by parents and relatives; reports and opinions from nurses, technicians, and other doctors; hospital records; and imaging studies. Most of these facts and data would have been admissible in evidence under common law, but only with the expenditure of substantial time in producing and examining various authenticating witnesses.[8] Today, the trial judge simply determines whether these types of information are "of a type reasonably relied upon" and are sufficiently related to the facts of the case.[9]

Expert testimony is not required in some malpractice cases. Under the "common knowledge" doctrine, there is no need for expert testimony when the physician's negligence occurred in so gross a manner that it is patently evident to a lay jury. For example, a patient who underwent a mastectomy on the wrong breast or amputation of the incorrect leg does not require the testimony of an expert witness to persuade the jury that the action constitutes malpractice.[10]

Limitations

An expert witness must testify as to what the "profession as a whole" regards as acceptable practice, not what he or she would have done in the same situation. As one court noted,[11] "The applicable standard of care is that employed by the medical profession generally and not what one individual doctor thought was advisable and would have done under the same circumstances." Indeed, it ruled that questions aimed at determining how the expert personally would have elected to treat the patient are irrelevant both on direct and cross-examination, even for purposes of impeachment.[12]

Expert witnesses are not permitted to offer legal conclusions, though they may render an opinion on an "ultimate issue of fact."[13] In practice, however, courts have been unable to draw a clear distinction between these ambiguous terms. An expert is precluded from expressing opinions about the credibility of other witnesses, since an evaluation of their trustworthiness is the function of the jury. Although the expert cannot tell the jury which witnesses to believe, expert testimony is not inadmissible simply because it may have the indirect effect of bolstering or attacking the credibility of another witness. A major limitation is that the testimony of an expert, as with any other witness, may be excluded "if its probative value (making the defendant more or less likely to be liable) is substantially outweighed by the danger of unfair prejudice, confusion of the issues, misleading the jury, or by considerations of undue delay, waste of time, or needless presentation of cumulative evidence." As the U.S. Supreme Court has noted, "expert evidence can be both powerful and quite misleading because of the difficulty in evaluating it," and thus the judge must be scrupulous in assuring that its probative value outweighs any negative effects.[14]

Qualifications

At common law, an expert testifying about the medical standard of care was required to demonstrate familiarity with the standard in the geographic location in which the defendant physician practiced. With medical care now generally standard throughout the United States, most jurisdictions have relaxed this requirement.

Physicians do not have to be board certified or even specialists in a particular field of medicine to render an opinion, as long as the allegations of negligence concern matters within their knowledge and observation[15] so that they are able to attest to the applicable standard of care and determine whether there is a causal connection between a violation of that standard and the injuries that resulted. Nevertheless, the American Medical Association's Code of Medical Ethics requires that medical experts should "have recent and substantive experience in the area in which they testify and should limit their testimony to their sphere of medical expertise."[16] The ACR provides more specific guidelines for the radiologist expert witness, recommending that the individual be an active practitioner of radiology, be certified by the American Board of Radiology or comparable organization, and be actively involved with the clinical practice of the subject matter of the case for at least three of the previous five years.[17] Moreover, the ACR guidelines mandate that the radiologist review the medical information in the case and the standards of practice prevailing at the time of the alleged malpractice, as well as be prepared to state the basis of the testimony presented and whether it is based on personal experience, specific clinical references, or generally accepted opinion in the specialty field. Failure to conform to any or all of these criteria may result in the expert's disqualification.[18]

From the standpoint of the defendant physician, the fact that the plaintiff's expert is not a member of the same specialty or subspecialty can be either beneficial or harmful. The jury may conclude that the plaintiff's case must be weak, since if it were strong there would have been no difficulty in finding a reputable expert witness in the same specialty as the defendant—a concept that the defense attorney will stress during cross-examination. Conversely, even though the plaintiff's expert may not be as well qualified, the expert may be an extremely persuasive witness who is more effective than one who was in the same specialty as the defendant.[19]

The determination of whether an expert witness is truly an expert qualified to render an opinion in a specific lawsuit is the exclusive province of the trial judge, whose decision on admissibility of testimony is virtually always affirmed on appellate review unless it is "manifestly erroneous"[20] or an "abuse of discretion."[21] As the U.S. Supreme Court stated, the judge is the ultimate gatekeeper as to who may testify at trial, based on "a preliminary assessment of whether the reasoning or methodology underlying the testimony is scientifically valid" and can be "applied to the fact in issue."[22] Once the judge has ruled that the expert testimony is admissible, it is up to the trier of fact (the jury, or the judge in a bench trial) to determine its credibility or weight. Consequently, the attorney who has retained the expert witness emphasizes his or her credentials, knowledge, and experience on direct examination, while the opposing attorney attacks the credibility of the expert witness through often aggressive and incisive cross-examination.[23]

A witness who is shown to be not truly an expert, or who testifies to opinions not based on a solid factual foundation, can have devastating consequences to the party that has retained the non-expert. If the jury deems one expert witness of the party as incompetent, it may well extend this view to all experts who testify on that party's behalf. In addition to losing the case, the party attempting to present an unqualified expert witness may be held liable for paying the legal fees of the opposing side, as well as be exposed to other judicial sanctions.[24]

Consequences of Disqualification to the Witness

The disqualification by the judge of a proposed expert witness as incompetent because of a lack of credentials or credibility may pose serious long-term consequences. As public records, trial and deposition transcripts are easily available to both plaintiff and defense attorneys who are searching for expert witnesses. Being judicially labeled as unqualified or incompetent may make it virtually impossible for an individual to testify as an expert in a future trial. In the federal court system, potential expert witnesses must provide a listing of other cases in which the witness has testified as an expert at trial or deposition within the preceding four years. This is not a requirement in all state courts, but attorneys in any court are allowed to request similar information. If the individual is nevertheless selected as an expert, the opposing attorney may discover the prior judicial notice of incompetence and use it to savagely attack the credibility of the expert witness at trial.[25]

Proper Behavior of an Expert Witness

Ideally, expert witnesses should be honest, unbiased seekers after truth and well-prepared regarding the facts and issues of the case; they should not be advocates or partisans of one side in the legal proceeding. Most physician experts try to be objective and fair; unfortunately, a few unscrupulous individuals fail to demonstrate such virtues, caring little for the truth and trying to deceive the members of the jury.[26]

It is essential that expert witnesses be consistent in their testimony throughout the legal proceeding. Defense experts who testify that the defendant's missing a lesion did not constitute a deviation from the standard of care, but then admit that they would have identified it and insisted that their medical students report it, destroys the credibility of their opinion.[27] From a medical-legal perspective, when asked whether one would personally have made the diagnosis, a better response might be: "I do not know; although I can see the abnormality in retrospect, I cannot say whether I would have seen it prospectively on the initial radiologic study."[28] Similarly, testimony by expert witnesses that a defendant radiologist was not required to telephone the referring physician about a new and expected finding loses its effect if they admit that they personally would have done so.[29]

Radiologists should always be careful to be absolutely truthful when responding under oath to all questions posed to them by attorneys. Statements regarding credentials or experience, as well as opinions regarding particular radiologic practices, that are rendered in one case can easily be obtained by the opposing attorney in a subsequent legal proceeding. The credibility of an expert witness can be destroyed during cross-examination if the opposing lawyer can show that he or she made contradictory or inconsistent statements or opinions about similar circumstances in a different lawsuit.[30]

It is unconscionable for expert witnesses to unexpectedly hedge or reverse their opinions during trial, since the party calling them has relied on what they had expressed previously. Radiology experts who feel compelled to change an opinion or withdraw from a case should immediately inform the attorney who retained them so that there is ample opportunity to secure an adequate replacement.[31]

"Reasonable Degree of Medical Certainty" Standard

An expert witness is usually asked whether the conduct of the defendant breached the standard of care "to a reasonable degree of medical certainty." In most cases, physicians cannot testify that their opinion is given with absolute scientific precision. However, there is general agreement that the opinion of an expert that his or her conclusion is merely "possible" does not constitute persuasive legal evidence. Courts differ as to the precise meaning of "a reasonable degree of medical certainty." To be legally credible, the opinion of an expert witness must be stated at least in terms of "probably" or "more likely than not." This indicates that the opinion is not mere conjecture, which would be no more valid than the jury's own speculation as to what is or is not possible.[32]

Practical Tips for the Radiology Expert Witness

Expert witnesses should remain unbiased and dispassionate. When asked whether the defendant radiologist did or did not breach the standard of care, expert witnesses should state their opinions as firmly as possible, within a "reasonable degree of medical certainty." They should answer each question fully, but not be verbose or offer irrelevant information. Although the role of expert witnesses are to aid the judge or jury in understanding technical medical aspects of the case, they should never appear condescending or pedantic, a style that tends to alienate the trier of fact.[33]

Ethical Considerations

Most jurisdictions do not permit the payment of a contingency fee to an expert witness. The American Bar Association Model Code of Professional Responsibility includes a disciplinary rule that states: "A lawyer shall not pay, offer to pay, or acquiesce in the payment of compensation to a witness contingent upon the content of his testimony or the outcome of the case."[34] This is eminently reasonable in view of the requirement that an expert witness be unbiased and not adopt a partisan position. Moreover, a lawyer in a civil proceeding is generally prohibited from making an *ex parte* contact with the opposing party's expert witness.[35]

Adverse Consequences of Being an Expert Witness

Some radiologists refuse to be expert witnesses because they are afraid of the possible adverse consequences of their testifying in court. In general, an expert witness is granted immunity from being sued for any opinion expressed in a judicial proceeding, since courts are convinced that without such immunity witnesses might not testify truthfully lest they themselves be sued in retaliation. Nevertheless, courtroom immunity does not extend to an expert witness who lies under oath. The commission of perjury can expose a witness to criminal prosecution, which upon conviction can result in a substantial fine and/or imprisonment.[36] False statements made by a witness, especially if related to his or her qualifications, can even lead the judge to declare a mistrial.[37] The American Medical Association is working with state medical societies to develop disciplinary measures that can be taken against physician expert witnesses who provide fraudulent testimony.[38]

Protecting the Radiologist from Being Falsely Accused by an Expert Witness[39]

A radiologist defendant in a malpractice suit should carefully scrutinize the curriculum vitae, affidavits, other documents, and testimony of any expert witness retained by the attorney for the plaintiff. Any inconsistency or inaccuracy in this material should be immediately brought to the attention of the defense lawyer. Although there may be an honest difference of opinion concerning whether the defendant radiologist has breached the standard of care, any opinion that has no reasonable basis for support or is based on facts not presented in the case may be grounds for asking the court to disqualify the witness.

Whenever possible, the defendant radiologist should attend the depositions of the radiology expert witnesses retained by the plaintiff's attorney. The presence of a knowledgeable defendant radiologist may prevent the expert witness from being tempted to exaggerate or overstate an opinion regarding any alleged breach of the standard of care. Moreover, the defendant radiologist can assist the defense attorney in formulating questions that may seriously challenge the basis of the opinion of the expert witness.

Endnotes

1 Boumil MM, Elias CE. *The Law of Medical Liability*. St. Paul, MN: West Publishing, 1995:36–38.
2 Ibid., 41–42.
3 Ibid., 38.
4 Berlin L. On being an expert witness. *AJR* 1997;168:607–610.
5 Dickey NW, Burkhart JH, Chisholm WS, et al. Recent opinions of the council on ethical and judicial affairs. *JAMA* 1986;256:2241.
6 Federal Rules of Evidence. 702.
7 Fed. R. Evid. 703.
8 Notes of Advisory Committee on 1972 Proposed Rules, Fed. R. Evid. 703.
9 Piorkowski JD. Medical testimony and the expert witness. In: Sanbar SS, Gibofsky A, Firestone MH, et al (eds). *Legal Medicine, 5th ed.* St. Louis, Mosby, 2001, pgs 98–99.

10 Boumil MM, Elias CE. *The Law of Medical Liability*. St. Paul, MN: West Publishing, 1995:44–46.

11 *Johnson v Riverdale Anesthesia Associates*, 563 S.E.2d 431 (Ga, 2002).

12 *Legal Medicine Q & A*. Schaumburg, IL: American College of Legal Medicine, 2003;2:2.

13 Federal Rules of Evidence. 704.

14 Piorkowski JD. Medical testimony and the expert witness. In: Sanbar SS, Gibofsky A, Firestone MH, et al (eds). *Legal Medicine, 5th ed*. St. Louis, Mosby, 2001, pgs 100–101.

15 *Jones v O'Young et al*, 607 NE2d 224 (Ill 1992).

16 American Medical Association Council on Ethical and Judicial Affairs. *Code of Medical Ethics, 9.07, Medical Testimony*. Chicago: American Medical Association, 1997:148–149.

17 American College of Radiology. *Digest of Council Actions, section II, K1, Testimony*. Reston, VA: American College of Radiology, 1998:128–129.

18 Berlin L, Williams DM. When an expert witness is not an expert. *AJR* 2000;174:1215–1219.

19 Berlin L. The deep pocket. *AJR* 2000;175:1243–1247.

20 *Salem v United States*, 370 U.S. 31, 35 (1962).

21 *General Electric Company v Joiner*, 522 U.S. 136, 118 S.Ct. 512, 515 (1997).

22 *Daubert v Merrell Dow Pharmaceuticals*, 509 US 579 (1993).   NO hyphen

23 Berlin L, Williams DM. When an expert witness is not an expert. *AJR* 2000;174:1215–1219.

24 Ibid.

25 Ibid.

26 Berlin L. On being an expert witness. *AJR* 1997;168:607–610.

27 *Gable v Mansfield General Hospital et al*. Ohio App LEXIX 6102, 1995. LEXIS

28 Berlin L. On being an expert witness. *AJR* 1997;168:607–610.

29 Ibid.

30 Berlin L, Williams DM. When an expert witness is not an expert. *AJR* 2000;174:1215–1219.

31 Berlin L. On being an expert witness. *AJR* 1997;168:607–610.

32 Piorkowski JD. Medical testimony and the expert witness. In: Sanbar SS, Gibofsky A, Firestone MH, et al (eds). *Legal Medicine, 5th ed*. St. Louis, Mosby, 2001, pg 102.

33 Berlin L. On being an expert witness. *AJR* 1997;168:607–610.

34 ABA Model Code DR 7-109(C).

35 Piorkowski JD. Medical testimony and the expert witness. In: Sanbar SS, Gibofsky A, Firestone MH, et al (eds). *Legal Medicine, 5th ed*. St. Louis, Mosby, 2001, pg 104.

36 Berlin L. On being an expert witness. *AJR* 1997;168:607–610.
37 *Prochazka v Barrett*, Fresno County (CA) Superior Court, case No. 454378-1, 1993.
38 Berlin L, Williams DM. When an expert witness is not an expert. *AJR* 2000;174:1215–1219.
39 Ibid.

6
Countersuits

In medical malpractice, a countersuit is an action brought by a physician against the physician's former patient (the plaintiff in the original malpractice action) and the patient's attorney.[1] The countersuit movement began in the mid-1970s with enthusiastic support by the medical profession in response to the dramatic rise in medical malpractice suits, many of which were perceived as lacking substantial merit.[2] However, the courts have rejected almost all countersuits, primarily because of the strong public policy interest in ensuring that injured parties have free and open access to the judicial system, as well as the fear that allowing countersuits would have a chilling effect on an injured party's ability to seek legal redress.[3]

Possible Causes of Action

Physicians have employed numerous common-law legal theories in their attempts to countersue patients and their attorneys for what the physicians have considered to be frivolous lawsuits. The most popular has been *malicious prosecution*, alleging that the patient-plaintiff wrongly initiated a civil lawsuit. This cause of action requires that the physician prove that the patient and attorney filed a malpractice lawsuit without probable cause and with legal malice (ill will is not required; lack of a reasonable belief in the likelihood of success may be sufficient); that the lawsuit eventually terminated in the physician's favor (jury verdict for the defendant, voluntary dismissal by the patient, or involuntary dismissal by the court, but not termination solely on procedural grounds); and that the physician suffered "special damages."[4] In some courts, "special damages" requires arrest or imprisonment, seizure of property, or some injury different from that ordinarily sustained by malpractice defendants; other courts expand this requirement to include harm to professional reputation, expenses incurred in defending the lawsuit, emotional distress, and loss of income during a trial.[5]

Abuse of process is the misuse of an otherwise legal procedure—the filing of a groundless malpractice suit not for the purpose for which it is designed, but rather for an ulterior motive such as to coerce a nuisance settlement. Suits based on this theory are rarely successful because of the difficult in proving this improper motivation. Some countersuits have been based on *defamation*, the idea that an unfounded suit attacks the professional reputation of the defendant physician. This cause of action also fails in virtually all cases, because of an underlying privilege that protects oral and written statements made in the course of judicial pro- ceedings. The threat of defamation lawsuits would have a chilling ef- fect on access to the courts and on honest testimony, and thus would be contrary to the public interest in the free and independent operation of the courts.[6] In rare instances, however, lawyers for plaintiffs have made such inflammatory statements attacking the defendant physician that the courts have awarded damages. Though recognizing the duty of an attorney to be a zealous advocate, one court observed: "In representing their clients, lawyers are expected to use the legitimate sidearms of a warrior. It is only when a lawyer uses the dagger of an assassin that he should be subjected to discipline or to personal liability."[7]

A final cause of action is to countersue a plaintiff's attorney for professional *negligence*, alleging that the attorney failed to investigate adequately the medical facts of the case in advance of filing a malprac- tice lawsuit. However, courts have consistently held that an attorney owes no duty to any party other than one's client, unless that third party was intended to benefit from the attorney's actions. "In the usual medi- cal malpractice case, an attorney owes a duty to the client (the patient) to zealously represent him or her and to prosecute the claim. Requiring a concurrent duty to a physician not to file an unjustified suit would create a conflict of interest between attorney and client, denying the latter a right to effective counsel and free access to the courts."[8]

What Should a Radiologist Do If Subjected to an Unjustified Suit?[9]

The probability of a physician prevailing in a countersuit "ranges from nil to extremely low." One prominent radiologist, who had previously been subjected to an unjustified suit, strongly urges his colleagues who have been sued and found not liable to "forsake thoughts of retaliation or revenge seeking and get on with their professional lives." They "should be consoled with the knowledge that the American legal system has worked effectively and fairly," noting that the plaintiff and attorney filing a losing malpractice suit have come out empty-handed after investing substantial time and money in their lost case.

Nevertheless, radiologists should consider legal action against plaintiffs' attorneys who have acted in an "unreasonable, irresponsible, or vexatious manner." Federal and many state courts will impose sanctions on such attorneys, as well as assess them for damages for courts costs and the attorneys' fees of physician-defendants who have been victimized by such deplorable behavior.

Finally, defendant-radiologists who consider the charges unfair should control their feelings of anger and despair and instead resolve to do all they can to support their own attorneys in preparing and making a thorough and vigorous defense.

Endnotes

1 Lee BH. Countersuits by health care providers. In: Sanbar SS, Gibofsky A, Firestone MH, et al (eds). *Legal Medicine, 5th ed.* St. Louis, Mosby, 2001, pg 186.

2 Berlin L. Countersuing plaintiffs and their attorneys who have sued for malpractice. *AJR* 1997;168:1153–1156.

3 Lee BH. Countersuits by health care providers. In: Sanbar SS, Gibofsky A, Firestone MH, et al (eds). *Legal Medicine, 5th ed.* St. Louis, Mosby, 2001, pg 191.

4 Curran WJ. Retaliatory actions in malpractice: doctors against lawyers and patients. *N Engl J Med* 1981;304:211–222.

5 Berlin L. Countersuing plaintiffs and their attorneys who have sued for malpractice. *AJR* 1997;168:1153–1156.

6 Lee BH. Countersuits by health care providers. In: Sanbar SS, Gibofsky A, Firestone MH, et al (eds). *Legal Medicine, 5th ed.* St. Louis, Mosby, 2001, pgs 188–189.

7 *Nelson v Miller et al.,* 607 P2d 438 (Kan 1980).

8 Lee BH. Countersuits by health care providers. In: Sanbar SS, Gibofsky A, Firestone MH, et al (eds). *Legal Medicine, 5th ed.* St. Louis, Mosby, 2001, pg 189.

9 Berlin L. Countersuing plaintiffs and their attorneys who have sued for malpractice. *AJR* 1997;168:1153–1156.

7
Alternative Dispute Resolution[1]

Resolving medical disputes using the formal adjudication process of court litigation is time-consuming and expensive and may not suit the needs of the parties. This has led to the increasing popularity of alternative dispute resolution (ADR) procedures, each of which has important strengths and limitations.

Limitations of Formal Adjudication

Use of the court system to resolve disputes precludes a "win-win" result. Since a decision is generally rendered for one party or the other, the resolution is mutually exclusive (i.e., one party wins and one party loses). Other limitations of formal adjudication include: "(1) the involuntary nature of the process (i.e., one party may be forced into adjudication by another party); (2) the imposition of a decision by a third-party, neutral decision maker with no specialized knowledge of the subject matter of the dispute; (3) the use of a formal process as determined by rigid rules not designed by the parties; (4) the existence of an adversarial system in which each party presents proofs and arguments (in a majority of cases via attorneys) and each party attempts to discredit the other party's proofs and arguments; and (5) the dispute process occurs and the conflict is resolved in a mandated public forum." The two most common alternative dispute resolution procedures to avoid these limitations are mediation and arbitration.

Mediation

Mediation is a process by which a neutral third party assists disputing parties in *negotiating* a resolution. The mediator merely assists the parties and has no formal power to impose any outcome upon them.

Generally selected by the two parties, the mediator usually does not evaluate their individual legal rights but merely facilitates communication between them. The mediation process is informal; the only rules are those imposed by the parties themselves or by the mediator in an attempt to improve communication. For example, it may be agreed that neither party will interrupt while the other is speaking. Mediation is a voluntary process; once entered into, however, the agreement to abide by the mediated decision is generally enforced by private contract law.

The major advantages of mediation include the private nature of the process and the confidentiality of the results. The focus is on improving communications between the parties so as to identify common interests, goals, and needs, which, it is hoped, will result in a mutually acceptable resolution of the conflict. In the absence of rigid legal rules, the parties can suggest creative and flexible solutions to address their specific concerns. However, if the mediator does not recognize situations in which unique party goals outweigh the joint benefits identified, the process may be frustrating, wasting the time and resources of both parties and mediator and ultimately requiring resolution by formal adjudication.

Arbitration

Arbitration is a formalized system of dispute resolution in which parties present proofs and arguments to a neutral third party, who is empowered to impose a *binding decision* upon them. At times there are multiple arbitrators, typically one selected by each party with these two choosing a third. The process is less formal that a judicial trial and the rules of evidence are not as rigidly applied.

A major advantage of arbitration is that the parties can select as decision makers one or more individuals with specialized expertise relating to the conflict. The arbitrated decision is final, the dispute proceedings and the decision itself are private, the parties determine the procedural rules and an objective standard for decision, and the cost for resolving the dispute (in time and money) is substantially less than with formal adjudication. Agreements to arbitrate are specifically enforceable according to both state and federal law, and courts have the power to declare in contempt a party failing to abide by an arbitration decision.

Alternative Dispute Resolution in Medical Malpractice

Alternative dispute resolution, especially arbitration, has been championed by some as an ideal method to resolve malpractice claims because of its reduced cost, the involvement of an informed decision maker, and a reduction in the emotional trauma that results from formal adjudication. Moreover, it enables plaintiffs with "minor" injuries to have their claims heard, and it may reduce frivolous malpractice cases. However, there are some significant negatives with this approach. As a voluntary process, it requires that all parties and attorneys agree to participate; however, in many cases one of the parties may believe that a jury trial offers a better chance of success. Defendants may be reluctant to participate because any payment to end the dispute will be reported to the National Practitioner Data Bank.

Despite these limitations, many institutional health care providers and managed care organizations in their contractual agreements now use mandatory arbitration to resolve any patient care disputes. Courts have consistently rejected patient challenges to mandatory arbitration clauses. However, some states have enacted safeguards to protect patients from what they perceive as the unfair advantages of managed care organizations that have extensive experience in this form of dispute resolution. For example, California courts have held that arbitrators must exercise good faith in all adjudication procedures, including disclosure of previous relationships with a party in the dispute. Moreover, managed care organizations are prohibited from unduly delaying arbitration procedures.

Endnotes

1 Liang BA. Alternative dispute resolution and application to medical disputes.In: Sanbar SS, Gibofsky A, Firestone MH, et al (eds). *Legal Medicine, 5th ed*. St. Louis, Mosby, 2001, pgs 50-54.

8
Criminal Prosecution[1]

Criminal prosecution of physicians has historically been uncommon, with most of the charges relating to allegations of insurance (including Medicare and Medicaid) fraud, sexual abuse of patients, or illegal use of prescription or controlled substances. In recent years, however, there has been a marked increase in criminal prosecutions of physicians for "reckless endangerment."

When and under what circumstances can a charge of medical malpractice be escalated to an accusation of criminal conduct? A person whose behavior is "grossly negligent" may be liable for involuntary manslaughter if his or her conduct results in the accidental death of another person. This requires conduct that is more than "ordinary negligence" (a "mere mistake of judgment") and rises to what can be termed "reckless"—a "gross lack of competency or gross inattention, or wanton indifference to the patient's safety, which may arise from gross ignorance of the science of medicine and surgery or through gross negligence, either in the application and selection of remedies, lack of proper skills in the use of instruments, and failure to give proper attention to the patient"that exposed the victim to a substantial danger of serious bodily harm or death. The fact that the patient consented to a specific treatment or operation is no defense to a criminal action against the physician.[2]

An intriguing question is whether a radiologist performing an excretory urogram in a patient with acute flank pain and suspected ureteral stone could be convicted of a criminal offense if the patient died of an anaphylactic reaction to intravenous contrast. Given the small, but definite, risk of adverse reaction and the fact that noncontrast computed tomography has essentially replaced excretory urography for this clinical indication, one could argue that the radiologist was reckless in unnecessarily exposing the patient to a known risk.

The individual factor that appears to figure most prominently in the decision to bring a criminal prosecution for medical negligence is the failure to provide appropriate follow-up care. Although the defendant physician may not have acted with "evil intent," he or she may face prosecution and even conviction if the actions appear to be those of a doctor who was careless, irresponsible, or indifferent to the welfare of the patient (i.e., "didn't give a damn!").[3]

A radiologist who receives any official or indirect information that a criminal investigation has been undertaken concerning his or her professional activities should immediately retain an attorney knowledgeable in criminal defense. Often an early response or even a personal appearance by the radiologist, if allowed, may satisfy an investigator or prosecutor and preempt a full-fledged and costly procedure. Radiologists subjected to criminal prosecution for what they perceive to be unjustified reasons should vigorously attempt to enlist the assistance of their state medical society, branch of the American College of Radiology, and any other professional organization that has the capability to provide legal and/or financial resources.

Endnotes

1 Eisenberg RL, Berlin L. When does malpractice become manslaughter? *AJR* 2002;179:331-335.
2 Twardy S. Crimes by health care providers. In: Sanbar SS, Gibofsky A, Firestone MH, et al (eds). *Legal Medicine, 5th ed.* St. Louis, Mosby, 2001, pg 172.
3 Filkins JA. "With no evil intent:" the criminal prosecution of physicians for medical negligence. *J Legal Med* 2001;22:467-499.

9
Professional Liability Insurance

Insurance protects the individual against the risk of loss by distributing the burden of losses over a large number of people, based on the law of averages. In medical practice, professional liability insurance is a contract in which the physician pays a specific premium to the insurance company or carrier, which in turn agrees to pay a party injured or harmed by the negligence of that physician the sum awarded by a trier of fact (judge, jury, or arbitration panel) or by settlement to compensate for the losses resulting from the injury. Like other insurance providers, medical liability carriers have a duty to act in good faith, which includes the requirement to defend the insured throughout all phases of the judicial process.[1]

Insurance Contracts

Most radiologists never read their professional liability insurance contracts at the time of purchase, only looking at them after a malpractice action has been filed against them. The essence of the insurance contract is an attempt to define those losses that are covered by the agreement and those that are excluded. It typically is written in tortured legal prose that has a readability index indicating that it is less understandable than Einstein's theory of relativity![2] Nevertheless, it is essential that radiologists have a reasonable understanding of the extent and limitations of prospective liability insurance contracts before purchasing malpractice policies, which generally represent the most important and expensive outlay that they make in their professional careers.[3]

Occurrence Versus Claims-Made Policies[4]

There are two basic types of professional liability insurance policies: occurrence and claims-made. *Occurrence* policies cover claims of alleged malpractice occurring during the policy period, regardless of when the lawsuit was filed or when the insurer was notified of the claim. *Claims-made* policies cover only claims of alleged malpractice reported during the policy period, regardless of when the service that is the basis of the claim was rendered.

If a radiologist maintains a liability insurance policy with the same company during his or her entire professional life, there is little difference in actual coverage between the occurrence and claims-made policies that are offered today. However, the distinction between these insurance products can have profound effects when a radiologist changes policies or retires.

Until the late 1970s, most policies were of the occurrence type. However, since the injuries resulting from medical malpractice may not become apparent for years after the incident (and substantially after the paid policy period), it was difficult for the insurance companies to accurately calculate the premium for risks. With inflation and spiraling jury awards, insurance companies sustained significant losses. Consequently, the vast majority of professional liability insurance companies shifted to claims-made policies, which precluded them from responsibility for claims that arose after the expiration of the policy and thus enabled them to calculate premiums with more prevision.

Tail and Nose Policies[5]

It is critical to remember that the event that triggers coverage in a claims-made policy is the formal *notification* of the company by the insured that a lawsuit has been filed, not the official filing of the malpractice action. Therefore, a claim is considered to exist only on the date that it is first reported by the insured to the company; if the radiologist fails to report a claim before the termination of a claims-made policy, even if due to reasonable lack of knowledge of the existence of the suit, the court deems that no timely claim has been made. To prevent the potentially devastating consequences of a gap when no insurance coverage is in effect when a physician switches from one claims-made policy to another, insurance companies offer optional plans to protect radiologists from alleged acts of malpractice committed either before the policy becomes active or after it expires.

"Tail insurance" is an amendment to a policy that provides that all claims arising from actions that occurred during the term of a claims-made policy are covered regardless of when they are reported (assuming that they are otherwise covered under the terms and conditions of the policy). In effect, this amendment puts these claims on an occurrence basis. Conversely, a "prior acts endorsement" ("nose insurance") provides coverage before the commencement date of a claims-made policy. "If a radiologist is applying for professional liability insurance for the first time, or if he or she has been practicing under an occurrence policy, the retroactive date of a claims-made policy corresponds to the date that the policy goes into effect…. A physician who changes from one claims-made policy to another and who wants continuous insurance protection must purchase either tail coverage from the first carrier or nose coverage from the second carrier."

Mandatory Insurance Requirements

According to the Joint Commission on Accreditation of Health Care Organizations, a hospital may require that all applicants for staff membership demonstrate evidence of adequate professional liability insurance. Some state laws permit hospitals to add mandatory insurance coverage requirements to their medical staff bylaws. Courts have consistently upheld these requirements as protecting the financial health of hospitals.[6] Having all physicians covered by malpractice insurance allows the hospital to save money on its own coverage (thus theoretically enabling it to provide patient care at lower cost), protects other staff physicians against liability for the malpractice of an uninsured physician on the staff, and ensures that each physician is able to contribute toward the cost of defense (and any subsequent adverse judgment) if the hospital were joined in a lawsuit against a staff physician.[7]

Amount of Insurance Coverage

Virtually all hospitals require that staff physicians maintain a minimum amounts of insurance coverage—usually $1 million for a single incident and $3 million for all alleged acts of malpractice committed within a one-year period. Because of the steady increase in multimillion dollar verdicts and settlements, some radiologists have decided to obtain coverage in excess of that required for hospital membership. Whether to purchase extra insurance may depend on the type of practice. For hospital-based radiologists named as a primary defendant in a medical malpractice suit, it is likely that other parties (hospital, referring physician, partners of the radiologist) will also be included as codefendants. The combined insurance policies of these multiple defendants should cover even the largest awards. Conversely, a radiologist practicing in a private office setting has a greater chance of being named the sole defendant and thus should consider purchasing extra insurance, though if this amount is substantially greater than that of one's referring physicians the radiologist may fall into the trap of being the "deep pocket" (see below).[8]

Radiologists should purchase professional liability insurance only from reputable companies legally authorized to conduct business in their state. They should ask colleagues who are already insured with the potential company whether it has handled previous malpractice claims in a prompt, efficient, and physician-friendly manner.[9] Never buy insurance solely on the basis of the premium charged.

The Deep Pocket

According to the doctrine of *joint and several liability*, defendants found liable in a malpractice lawsuit share among themselves the total amount awarded to the plaintiff. However, since not all parties have the same coverage, the defendants with the greatest amounts of insurance—the "deep pockets"—may find themselves paying the most money. An even worse situation occurs when a primary nonradiologist defendant in a malpractice action carries insufficient insurance. A radiologist may be named as a co-defendant despite being only minimally involved in the case, simply because he or she carries a large amount of insurance and is viewed as the deep pocket. "An effective strategy used by plaintiffs' attorneys in a situation of this type is to settle out-of-court with the underinsured primary defendant physician, and then to proceed to trial with the radiologist as the only defendant. Because a radiologist is responsible for his or her negligence even if another physician involved in the case has committed an act of greater negligence, the radiologist may thus wind up paying the lion's share of indemnification." Therefore, radiologists with more insurance than their clinical colleagues run the risk of having to pay a greater percentage of any damage award, or of being dragged in as a secondary codefendant in a case in which they would not otherwise have been named if they had less insurance coverage.[10]

Defense of Malpractice Claims

Although hired by the insurance company, the defense attorney in a malpractice suit has a duty to be a zealous advocate of the best interests of the radiologist. The requirement to balance the needs of both of these parties can lead to a conflict of interest, especially when the radiologist and insurance company have disparate views on whether to settle a case. If dissatisfied with the quality or tactics of the defense attorney assigned to the case, a radiologist should immediately complain in writing to the insurance carrier; if necessary, the radiologist should formally request that the company provide a different attorney. The insurance company generally will comply with such a request, since failure to do so could make it legally vulnerable to a charge of bad faith for not appropriately considering the interests of the radiologist-insured.[11]

Should a radiologist subject to a malpractice suit retain a personal attorney in addition to the defense counsel supplied by the insurance carrier? According to Berlin, in most cases, this is an unnecessary expense since the primary duty of the defense attorney is to the physician-insured, rather than to the insurance company that is paying the bill. However, the radiologist should consider retaining a personal attorney in the infrequent occasion in which there is a dispute between the physician and the insurer "(a) regarding availability or extent of coverage; (b) regarding consideration of a settlement without consent of the physician in violation of policy terms; or (c) if there is a likelihood of a settlement or verdict in excess of maximum insurance coverage."[12]

Settlement of Lawsuits

In general, liability insurance contracts give the insurer absolute authority to settle claims within the policy limits, in accord with the doctrine that the law favors settlement without recourse to litigation. Nevertheless, most medical malpractice policies contain a clause that requires the insurer to obtain the consent of the insured before settling with a plaintiff.[13] The reason for this distinction is that "claims arising out of professional negligence or misconduct do not only result in judgments or settlements against professionals, but also may affect the professional's reputation and thereby his future livelihood."[14] Settlements of malpractice suits (and jury verdicts against defendant physicians) are reported to the National Practitioner Data Bank, which was established to facilitate state and hospital awareness of physicians who have been disciplined in one state and then move to another state and become licensed.[15] The Data Bank also includes any restriction or other penalties imposed by governmental agencies on a physician's medical license, as well as any suspension or revocation of hospital privileges. Because these are permanent records that are available to hospitals, insurance companies, and managed care organizations, an unfavorable report may have a detrimental impact on a physician's future ability to gain a state medical license, secure reasonably priced professional liability insurance, obtain hospital privileges, or be selected for a managed care contract.[16]

Consequently, "settlement of a malpractice suit, or acceptance of a compromise agreement arising from an investigation by a state licensing board or a hospital disciplinary committee, should be entered into with great caution and only if the radiologist believes, after consultation with an attorney, that no better alternative exists." Unless there is no hope, a radiologist should never "give in" and accept such a compromise agreement because of not wanting to spend the time and effort to resist it. Despite facile assurances that a settlement does not indicate any guilt, the opposite is usually true, since most governmental agencies and insurance companies deem a voluntary settlement to be just as strong an indication of wrongdoing as a jury verdict or decision by a fact-finding board. Therefore, whenever possible a radiologist sued for malpractice should always attempt to gain dismissal of the lawsuit or a verdict of nonliability.[17] Indeed, radiologists should select an insurance company with a reputation of not settling claims too quickly, being wary of companies that appear to be more concerned with protecting themselves than the insured physician.[18]

Nevertheless, radiologists should not unreasonably withhold consent to settle a hopeless case. By refusing a settlement offer against the advice of the insurance company, a radiologist could be held liable for payment of the additional funds if a jury later awards damages in excess of the sum for which the case could have been settled.[19]

At times, an insurance company may refuse to a settle a lawsuit even though the physician-insured has requested that it do so. This occurs most frequently when a patient who has sued a radiologist offers to settle for an amount at or near the upper the limits of the policy. The insurance company may feel that it has little to lose financially by going to court, while the radiologist wishes to avoid the emotional trauma and adverse media attention that would result from an open trial. When faced with such a situation, a radiologist should document in writing the request to settle. If a jury ultimately awards damages in excess of the insured's policy limits, the carrier may be held responsible for paying the entire award.[20] Moreover, the insurance carrier may be liable for "emotional distress and injury to business goodwill that [may] flow from the failure to settle," even if the radiologist did not suffer any financial loss.[21]

Endnotes

1 Zimmerly JG, Hubler JR. Health insurance and professional liability insurance. In: Sanbar SS, Gibofsky A, Firestone MH, et al (eds). *Legal Medicine, 5th ed.* St. Louis, Mosby, 2001, pgs 192–193.
2 Ibid., 196.
3 Berlin L. Professional liability insurance. *AJR* 1998;170:565–569.
4 Ibid.
5 Ibid.
6 Ibid.
7 *Stein v Tri-City Hospital Authority*, 384 SE.2d (GA App 1989).

8   Berlin L. The deep pocket. *AJR* 2000;175:1243–1247.

9   Berlin L. Professional liability insurance. *AJR* 1998;170:565–569.

10 Berlin L. The deep pocket. *AJR* 2000;175:1243–1247.

11 Berlin L. Professional liability insurance. *AJR* 1998;170:565–569.

12 Ibid.

13 Ibid.

14 *Saucedo v Winger*, 915 P2d 129 (Kan App 1996).

15 Zimmerly JG, Hubler JR. Health insurance and professional liability insurance. In: Sanbar SS, Gibofsky A, Firestone MH, et al (eds). *Legal Medicine, 5th ed*. St. Louis, Mosby, 2001, pg 207.

16 Berlin L. Consequences of being accused of malpractice. *AJR* 1997;169: 1219–1223.

17 Ibid.

18 Zimmerly JG, Hubler JR. Health insurance and professional liability insurance. In: Sanbar SS, Gibofsky A, Firestone MH, et al (eds). *Legal Medicine, 5th ed*. St. Louis, Mosby, 2001, pg 207.

19 Berlin L. Professional liability insurance. *AJR* 1998;170:565–569.

20 Ibid.

21 *Landow v. Medical Insurance Exchange of California*, 892 F Supp 239 (D Nev 1995).

10
Special Residency Issues

Insurance

Like all other physicians, radiology residents may be held liable for malpractice if they negligently cause injury to patients by breaching the standard of care. Some state courts have ruled that residents are held to a higher standard of medical care than that for general practitioners, but less than that for fully qualified members of the specialty.[1] Others have disagreed, declaring that "a resident who holds himself out as a specialist shall be held to the standard of skill expected of a specialist."[2] Even if the former viewpoint prevails in a given state, a radiology resident should not be lulled into a false sense of security regarding liability. "A court ruling that a resident is held to a lower standard of care than a fully trained specialist may mitigate the amount of damage assessed on the resident for patient injury and may expand the culpability of the resident's employer, but such a ruling will not relieve residents from the expense of defending themselves and participating financially in any verdict or settlement."[3]

Radiology residents usually take it for granted that professional liability insurance is provided for them by their residency programs. Nevertheless, they should be aware of the specific type of coverage and any policy exclusions that could lead to financial disaster. If a claims-made policy (see page 64) is in effect, it is critical that the resident make certain that tail coverage is provided by the residency program upon completion of the residency. If tail coverage is not provided, residents leaving the program will be uninsured for subsequent claims arising from their practice during residency. Most residency liability policies have certain restrictions or exclusions. The most common exclusion is for "moonlighting" activities. Although many residents supplement their income by practicing elsewhere at night or on weekends, almost all residency liability insurance policies do *not* cover these activities. Consequently, it is essential that residents who elect to moonlight investigate whether adequate insurance is provided by the health care facility where they will be working. If not, residents should purchase professional liability insurance for these "extracurricular" activities, lest they run the potentially devastating risk of being uninsured for claims resulting from moonlighting.[4]

Another insurance issue of concern for residents is known as "surcharging" or "experience rating." The widespread impression that the malpractice crisis has been caused by a small number of bad doctors has led some insurance companies and state commissioners to adopted plans that "assess points against a physician for the number of malpractice claims experienced, the outcome of the claims, and the amount paid on behalf of the physician. When a physician exceeds a certain point threshold, he or she is typically assessed an additional premium over and above the normal premium for that specialty." This may especially impact on residents, since it is common practice for plaintiffs' attorneys to file suit against all healthcare providers whose names appear in a plaintiff's medical chart. "A resident who has experienced a number of malpractice claims during residency should investigate the surcharging or experience-rating practices of prospective insurance carriers or states prior to going into private practice. The resident who neglects these inquiries may find that insurance is unavailable or prohibitively expensive."[5]

Special Liability Status[6]

Even though radiology residents are under supervision, as physicians licensed to practice medicine, they may be held individually liable for their actions. It is essential that residents (or their supervisors) inform patients of their status, lest they risk being exposed to a lawsuit for alleged fraud, deceit, misrepresentation, assault and battery, or lack of informed consent. Having a resident's status clearly indicated on a name tag is one way to address this issue. Any discussion of one's residency status with a patient should be documented in the medical record, as should the patient's decision whether to accept or refuse medical services from the resident.

Rather than have an inflated or unrealistic sense of their abilities, residents must be continually aware of the limits and extent of their training and expertise. When unsure of how to interpret a difficult study or perform a new procedure, a resident (like a fully trained radiologist) is obligated to seek assistance from one who is more experienced. "Courts have little sympathy when a physician attempts procedures or treatments that are beyond the scope of his or her knowledge and experience, no matter how well they are actually performed."

Endnotes

1 *Jistarri v Nappi*, 549 A2d 210 (PA App 1988).
2 *Valentine v Kaiser Foundation Hospital*, 194 Cal App2d 282 (Cal 1961).
3 Berlin L. Liability of the moonlighting resident. *AJR* 1998;171:565-567.
4 *Medical-Legal Issues for Residents in Radiology*. Reston, VA: American College of Radiology, 1994:3-5.
5 Ibid., 5.
6 Ibid., 13.

11
Reactions of Physicians Sued for Malpractice

Few events in a physician's career are as traumatic as a medical malpractice suit.[1] Each year in the United States, the tort system generates nearly one suit for every five physicians overall.[2] Physicians who are sued for malpractice experience a series of emotional responses that are both predictable and common. These are comparable to the stages of grieving described in literature, but involve additional responses unique to medicine.[3]

The initial shock after being notified that one is the object of a malpractice suit is followed by denial—some combination of the feelings that "This cannot be happening to me" and "Maybe this will go away." These early emotional stages can have catastrophic consequences to the defense of the lawsuit, since the physician may fail to file time-sensitive documents such as written answers to the complaint and interrogatories, which can result in adverse events including deemed admissions, stricken pleadings, or even default judgments.[4]

Shock and denial eventually lead to stages of anger and depression (see below). However, sued physicians also experience emotional trauma that has been reported to be unique to the medical-legal environment—isolation, shame, and fear.[5] Legal counsel generally cautions the physician not to discuss the case with anyone, fearing that such conversations could be used against the physician in court. Although this may be necessary and appropriate from the legal point of view, it tends to isolate the physician emotionally by magnifying feelings of having to cope alone with the situation and being unable to share the emotional burden with others.[6] In addition, physicians are particularly likely to feel ashamed about being sued, regardless of the merits of the case. The mere fact of being sued evokes feelings of unworthiness and inadequacy, often leading the physicians to doubt their own skills and capabilities, despite evidence that, paradoxically, superior physicians are the ones most often sued. Physicians often find themselves isolated from the support of both colleagues and family; spouses frequently describe sued physicians as being withdrawn, remote, and uncommunicative. Physicians who have been sued often experience intense fear as to the possible effect of the legal action on their career, reputation, and finances.[7]

Most sued physicians experience intense anger at the plaintiff, bewildered that their patients could have taken legal action after all the time and effort they had expended in attempting to provide them with the best medical care ("How could the patient do this to me when I worked so hard for him/her?"). They quickly realize that in malpractice allegations there is a strong correlation between the severity of the disability (not whether there has been negligence) and the outcome, engendering strong reactions from physicians who perceive this as an injustice in the system.[8]

Many physicians who have been sued for malpractice exhibit a cluster of symptoms associated with clinical depression, including insomnia, loss of appetite and energy, decreased libido, and moodiness. Others common manifestations include chronic headaches, irritability, feelings of constant inattention, and gastrointestinal distress. In one study, 16% of physicians experienced the onset or exacerbation of physical illness, most commonly coronary disease, hypertension, colitis, and duodenal ulcer.[9] In some physicians, a medical malpractice lawsuit may result in destructive behavior, such as the excessive use of alcohol, drug abuse, or even attempted suicide. "Because litigation runs a course that is often lengthy and unpredictable, there inevitably occurs an ebbing and recurrence of the symptoms, which are triggered by any new development in the case. Even the sight of an unopened envelope from the defense attorney or a call from the insurance company can cause an adrenaline rush for the sued physician."[10]

Supporting a Sued Radiologist

Whatever the outcome, virtually all physicians who have been sued agree that their lives are never quite the same again. Some are so devastated that they completely give up the practice of medicine.[11]

Nevertheless, there are positive steps that can be taken. Physicians who are being sued for malpractice should become actively involved in their defense. Enhancing the sense of gaining control can lessen frustration and the uncomfortable feeling of dependence. The sued physician can be invaluable in educating the defense attorney about the case by pointing out both its strengths and weaknesses, as well as aiding in devising strategies and selecting expert witnesses who may make the difference between winning and losing the case.[12] It is important for the sued physician to remember that 80% of all claims are closed in the doctor's favor.[13] Moreover, if a lawsuit goes to trial, chances are still four-to-one that the physician will be exonerated.[14]

Health permitting, it is valuable for a physician being sued for malpractice to engage in aggressive aerobic sports, such as handball and tennis. This not only improves the physician's physical condition, but also provides a socially acceptable method of venting tension and anger. Spending time teaching student and residents can serve to raise the defendant-physician's diminished sense of self-esteem.[15]

The chairperson of the medical group should make every effort to alleviate the sense of isolation suffered by physicians sued for malpractice by emphasizing that they are not alone. He or she should suggest a more flexible schedule, since a hectic workload can exacerbate the stress and anxiety generated by a lawsuit.[16] To help ease the personal and emotional trauma experienced by all doctors who are sued, one large physician organization in Texas has begun a program to provide peer support to physicians in this time of great need.[17] The development of similar support groups throughout the country would be extremely valuable to maintaining the emotional well-being of physicians who are subjected to malpractice lawsuits.

Endnotes

1 File AE. My malpractice case was literally a trial by fire. *Medical Economics*. March 19, 2001;78:57-58,61.
2 Anderson RE. Outcomes of medical-malpractice litigation. Correspondence. *N Engl J Med* 1997;336:1681.
3 Couch CE, Thiebaud S. Who supports physicians in malpractice cases? *The Physician Executive* March-April 2002;30-33.
4 Ibid.
5 Ibid.
6 Gorney M. Coping with bad news: the physician executive's role in a lawsuit. *The Physician Executive* March-April 2002;26-29.
7 Couch CE, Thiebaud S. Who supports physicians in malpractice cases? *The Physician Executive* March-April 2002;30-33.
8 Ibid.
9 Charles S, Kennedy E. *Defendant*. New York: Free Press, 1985.
10 Gorney M. Coping with bad news: the physician executive's role in a lawsuit. *The Physician Executive* March-April 2002;26-29.
11 Ibid.

12 Ibid.

13 *Medical Malpractice Claims Review*. Napa, CA: The Doctors' Company, 2000.

14 Gorney M. Coping with bad news: the physician executive's role in a lawsuit. *The Physician Executive* March-April 2002;26-29.

15 Ibid.

16 Ibid.

17 Couch CE, Thiebaud S. Who supports physicians in malpractice cases? *The Physician Executive* March-April 2002;30-33.

12
Role of the Radiologist-Defendant at Trial[1,2]

Full cooperation of the radiologist-defendant is essential at trial. He or she should plan on being present in the courtroom for every day of evidence, from the time of opening statements until closing arguments. The radiologist-defendant must arrange coverage for all clinical, academic, and administrative activities so as to be totally committed to the judicial proceedings. Absence of the defendant inevitably suggests to jurors that the radiologist is not sufficiently concerned about the case, because of either arrogance or guilt. Moreover, the radiologist plays a major role in assisting defense counsel in both cross-examination of plaintiff witnesses and in the direct examination of witnesses for the defense.

In the courtroom, the radiologist should look, act, and testify as a well-qualified physician. Prior to giving testimony, the radiologist must engage in intensive preparation. Direct examination by the defense attorney should be practiced in a courtroom-type setting, so that the radiologist is as comfortable as possible when actually on the stand. The radiologist should be subjected to a mock cross-examination in order to practice responding to expected questions from the plaintiff's attorney. When testifying, the radiologist should look at the members of the jury and speak to them "as if they were a small group of relatives at a family reunion." The radiologist's explanations should be clear and concise, never condescending, yet not filled with technical jargon that may be designed to impress the jury but will usually have the opposite effect by making them "alienated by a perceived sense of egotism."

It is essential for the radiologist-defendant to carefully review the deposition before trial. The plaintiff's attorney will use any testimony given in court that is inconsistent with or contradicts answers provided during the prior deposition to impugn the radiologist's credibility. If the radiologist is convinced that for some reason he or she must disagree with deposition testimony when on the stand, this should be carefully discussed with the defense attorney so that such disagreements can be appropriately explained to the satisfaction of the jury.

The radiologist should be certain that he or she fully understands the question of opposing counsel, asking for it to be repeated if necessary. Hypothetical questions ("Assume for a moment…") and those that must be answered either "yes" or "no" are potential pitfalls. If a hypothetical question concerns the plaintiff in the specific case, it is important for the radiologist to make it clear to the jury that the answer relates only to a hypothetical patient and not to the case at trial. In "yes-no" questions, especially if long and convoluted, the radiologist should answer in the negative if there is even a single word with which he or she disagrees. This forces the plaintiff attorney to either ask the reason for this negative response, which allows the radiologist to fully explain the answer, or to move on to a different question (blunting any impact of the previous one).

Whenever testifying, the radiologist should always remember the critical difference between an "error" and a "breach of the standard of care." An error is "an objective act," and it may be reasonable for the radiologist to admit making it, especially if it could only be seen in retrospect with the advantage of knowing the future course of the patient. However, the radiologist must never admit to a breach of the standard of care, for this is effectively an admission of negligence.

When not testifying, the radiologist-defendant should pay attention to the testimony and offer suggestions to the defense attorney whenever appropriate. The radiologist should remain composed and in control at all times, since he or she is always in view of the jury.

Endnotes

1 Petrek RF Jr, Slovis MR. The defendant in a malpractice suit: an integral part of the defense team. *Pediatr Radiol* 1998;28:905–912.
2 Berlin L. Failure to diagnose lung cancer: anatomy of a malpractice trial. *AJR* 2003;180:37–45.

13
Risk Management

As defined by the Joint Commission on Accreditation of Health Care Organizations (JCAHO), risk management encompasses "clinical and administrative activities that [health care organizations] undertake to identify, evaluate, and reduce the risk of injury and loss to patients, personnel, visitors, and [the organization] itself."[1] A successful risk management must be both reactive (to incidents that have already occurred) and proactive (to prevent future occurrences). Thus, risk management deals with "identification of legal risk, prioritization of identified risk, determination of proper organizational response to risk, management of recognized risk cases with the goal of minimizing risk (risk control), establishment of effective risk prevention, and maintenance of adequate risk financing."[2]

Radiologists should join all their medical colleagues in cooperating fully with health care facilities in designing and implementing an effective risk management program. "Rather than wait for a legal action, a record request, a patient complaint, or a billing dispute to initiate the process of risk identification," radiologists should immediately notify the risk management department whenever they encounter an "untoward or unusual incident." In some institutions, this may include the filling out of an "incident report form" detailing the radiologist's view of what transpired.[3] At times, skilled risk management personnel may be able to handle the situation so well at this stage that they preclude subsequent litigation.

Communication with Patients[4]

Although risk management is a complicated process, radiologists should never forget that the best (and simplest) way of avoiding malpractice lawsuits is proper communication with patients. Litigation is usually triggered by a bad outcome, but adverse events are substantially more likely to lead to lawsuits if there are problems in communication that have led to patient frustration and dissatisfaction. Therefore, developing positive relationships with patients and demonstrating sensitivity to their needs is not only good medical practice but also a superb method for minimizing the risk of liability.

From the initial encounter, radiologists should establish a good rapport with their patients. They should be sensitive to their personal characteristics, such as gender, culture, language, race, and social status, and thoughtfully ask how they wish to be addressed. By being aware of and understanding the patient's fear and anxieties, the radiologist can take positive steps to allay them and thus make the patient feel as comfortable as possible. Never forget that establishing good eye contact is valuable for effective communication. The radiologist should be "positive, caring, and respectful"; if an unexpected event should unfortunately occur, a sincere demonstration of "warmth, understanding, and concern [and immediate availability] can go a long way toward alleviating potential problems." The patient should be "treated as a mature, intelligent human being and dealt with honestly … as you or a member of your family would want to be treated." The goal is to have the patient perceive the radiologist as a trustworthy ally, dedicated to the patient's well-being. When explaining a procedure or treatment, the radiologist should allow the patient to share responsibility in decision making by disclosing all relevant facts, clearly explaining any alternatives and reservations, and answering all questions. The positive interaction between radiologists and patients established by such effective communication can substantially reduce the risk of malpractice suits.

Endnotes

1 Joint Commission on Accreditation of Health Care Organizations. *Accreditation Manual for Hospitals* 262 (JCAHO 1992).
2 Balsamo RR, Brown MD. Risk management. In: Sanbar SS, Gibofsky A, Firestone MH, et al (eds). *Legal Medicine, 5th ed.* St. Louis, Mosby, 2001, pg 212.
3 Ibid., 216.
4 *Medical-Legal Issues for Residents in Radiology.* Reston, VA: American College of Radiology, 1994:17–19.

Part II
The Missed Diagnosis: Overview

14
The Missed Diagnosis: Overview

When is an error simply an unfortunate mistake and when is it malpractice? Despite years of debate and numerous judicial proceedings, whether a missed radiographic diagnosis constitutes malpractice remains a vexing question without a practical answer.

Frequency of Errors

In the past few years, there have been alarming news reports of an unacceptably high frequency of medical errors. The publication of an Institute of Medicine report[1] stating that medical errors cause from 44,000 to 98,000 deaths each year in American hospitals shocked the public and resulted in banner headlines that doctors' mistakes "kill" almost 100,000 Americans annually. Some have questioned the accuracy of the study, noting that it includes many patients who were so ill that they would have died regardless of whether any errors were committed.[2] Furthermore, adverse events and medical errors do not necessarily imply that there has been physician negligence. Two studies have shown that negligence is responsible for adverse events in less than one third of cases.[3,4]

For more than a half century, numerous articles have documented that diagnostic errors occur in about 30% of cases.[5] Even higher miss rates have been reported in relation to the diagnosis of cancer in mammography[6] and chest radiography.[7] However, statistics from these carefully controlled retrospective studies do not reflect the actual error rates committed by radiologists in daily practice. They fail to account for the availability of clinical information, interaction with other physicians, and the fact that many imaging studies are normal.[8] A study[9] of the actual radiographic interpretations, most of which were normal, rendered in several community hospitals revealed only a 4.4% error rate—reasonably similar to the reported frequency of adverse events found in hospitalizations.[10,11]

Radiologists reading the same radiograph at different times disagree with themselves in up to 20% of cases.[12] Therefore, Berlin suggests that when asked by a referring physician the results of a specific examination, rather than answering, "I have read the film, and it is normal," it is preferable and more prudent to say, "I did read it as normal, but let's look at it again together." He adds, "A second look by the radiologist, with or without a referring physician or colleague, will occasionally reveal a radiographic finding that was initially overlooked."[13]

Causes of Errors

Radiologic errors may be cognitive—in which a perceived abnormality is misinterpreted due to lack of/incomplete knowledge or faulty reasoning/judgment—or perceptual, with the abnormality not even seen.[14] Another source of radiologic error relates to the technical factors of inadequate exposure or positioning.[15]

Incomplete Knowledge

In some cases, radiologists miss the correct diagnosis not because of an inability to perceive the abnormalities, but rather because of failure to recognize them due to lack (or lapse) of knowledge. Courts have held that radiologists are required to possess and apply "ordinary knowledge"—that which would be expected of those who are minimally qualified members of the specialty. It is not necessary for a radiologist to be as skilled or knowledgeable as the recognized experts in the field. Nevertheless, the legal definition of what constitutes "ordinary knowledge" has never been precisely spelled out. Although the radiologic establishment has long acknowledged subspecialization and recognizes board certification and Certificates of Added Qualification (CAQ) in certain subspecialties as objective measures of competence, in individual malpractice cases the courts have not yet recognized such subspecialties or achievements in radiology (or any other medical specialty) as criteria of whether a radiologist possessed "ordinary knowledge."[16]

Given the realities of radiology practice, it is unrealistic to expect that every imaging study will be interpreted by the best-qualified radiologist. Most departments have some radiologists with fellowship training and expertise who limit their practice to a specific subspeciality. However, when the primary subspecialist is unavailable, the area must be covered by a radiologist with less training and experience. Nevertheless, all radiologists must maintain a basic ordinary knowledge of the types of imaging studies they interpret. This is especially important after normal working hours, when a single radiologist may be on call for an entire group. It is critical that radiologists interpret only the studies for which they are confident that they possess sufficient knowledge. If a radiologist feels inadequate to interpret a particular study, it is essential to refer the examination to an associate with the proper qualifications, or at least to confer with a knowledgeable person before rendering an opinion.[17]

Errors in Judgment

Another cause for making an incorrect diagnosis despite observing the abnormalities is faulty reasoning—failure to appreciate the significance of a finding, which is often related to an inability to think of the various possibilities that could produce it. When interpreting imaging studies, it is essential that radiologists take significant time for deliberation and reflection. Rather than coming to a hasty conclusion, radiologists should make a conscious effort to ask themselves whether there are any reasonable diagnostic alternatives. Could an apparent artifact represent a true lesion? Could the smooth pulmonary nodule represent something other than a benign granuloma? Consultations with radiology colleagues and referring physicians before rendering final reports may be of value, for they may raise diagnostic possibilities not entertained by a single radiologist reading in isolation. The classic axiom, "If you do not think of it, you will not diagnose it" implies that radiologists must continually reinforce and expand their base of knowledge through reading the current scientific literature and attending continuing medical education programs. Radiologists must also recognize that personal experience may be limited and not a reliable predictor of the prevalence of a given medical condition, so that a diagnostic possibility should not be summarily dismissed simply because one has never seen it before.[18]

Errors in judgment do not automatically make a physician liable for malpractice. "If a doctor has given the plaintiff the benefit of his best judgment, assuming that judgment to be equal to that ordinarily used by a reasonably qualified doctor in similar cases, he is not liable for negligence, even if that judgment is erroneous.... [Although] other physicians may have handled the case differently, if a reasonably well-qualified doctor might have proceeded in the same manner as the defendant, [the doctor is not negligent]."[19] Unfortunately, the precise point where an error in judgment becomes negligence is unclear. "Negligence occurs not merely when there is an error, but when the degree of error exceeds an accepted norm."[20] Furthermore, "No inference of malpractice arises from the mere fact that there was an undesirable result.... The law does not make a physician an insurer of the best result of his treatment."[21] Ultimately, it is up to the trial judge or jury to determine whether a specific radiographic diagnostic error in judgment is one that could be made by a reasonably well-qualified radiologist (and thus within the standard of care), or whether it violated the standard of care and thus constituted an act of negligence.[22]

Perceptual Errors

Perceptual errors are by far the most common cause of radiologic misses, accounting for up to 80% of them. In many cases, radiologists who fail to detect an abnormality on the initial interpretation can readily see it in retrospect and are baffled as to why they missed the lesion in the first place.[23] The inability to detect a radiographic abnormality is often attributed to its subtlety or "poor conspicuity," defined as the ratio between the contrast enhancement of the lesion or edge relative to the surrounding tissues.[24] However, this cannot explain the mystery of how a radiologist can miss on first look a retrospectively obvious lung nodule, filling defect in the colon, bone lucency, or breast calcifications.[25]

Numerous studies have shown a statistically significant increase in the rate of true-positive readings when a relevant clinical history is provided. "There are at least two aspects of clinical information pertinent to radiographic inspection: (a) indication of specific locations for intensive evaluation; and (b) clues to search for specific abnormalities." In patients with trauma, the error rate in detecting subtle fractures is halved when localizing clues are provided. These data substantiate the radiologists' requests that referring physicians provide appropriate clinical information.[26]

The percentage of malpractice lawsuits alleging missed fractures in which the radiologist was not provided with adequate clinical information indicating the site of pathology is unknown. Nevertheless, it is clear that "implementation and strict enforcement of hospital and clinical protocols requiring that the request for radiologic services in orthopedic trauma include pertinent history of the injury could significantly reduce the number of radiologic interpretations resulting in litigation." A protocol requiring radiologists to seek the additional information only in cases that they believed were questionable would not be effective, since an experimental study demonstrated that false-negative interpretations of abnormal cases without location clues were made with a high level of confidence.[27] Several practical methods for improving access to localizing information have been suggested—having the technologist mark the exact site of tenderness with a small lead marker, and noting the absence of relevant clinical information on the official radiology report.[28]

The missed lung cancer has been the focus of extensive study. The generally accepted error rate for the detection of early lung cancer is 20% to 50%, and there has been little improvement over the past few decades.[29] One suggested underlying factor is faulty visual search patterns and inadequate search duration. The majority of obvious lung cancers are detected with flash viewing of the radiograph (0.2 second).[30] Although there is severe impairment of the detection of subtle lung cancers if the viewing time is reduced to less than 4 seconds,[31] prolonged viewing time is of little or no value. Within 10 seconds, the average radiologist will have studied 85% of the lung and detected all nodules that will be reported.[32] Prolonging the viewing time much further will not increase the number of true-positive readings, but will increase the number of false positives,[33] which can lead to unnecessary and costly diagnostic studies and even a needle or open biopsy of a nonexistent lesion.

Small contrast differences between a lung nodule and the surrounding area decrease the rate of detection, especially in poorly penetrated areas of the lung (subpleural, retrodiaphragmatic, retrocardiac, paramediastinal). Superimposed structures and the complexity of the area surrounding a nodule decrease lesion detection, especially in the apical and perihilar areas. End-on and overlapping vessels and ribs may simulate or camouflage a nodule, causing confusion and competing for the radiologist's attention. Poorly defined and speculated nodules, which are more difficult to detect than smooth ones, may be difficult or impossible to perceive until they become quite large. Improper viewing conditions can adversely affect the detection rate of lung nodules. Ideally, interpretation of radiographs should occur "in a calm environment free of constant interruption and time pressure"—a situation infrequently achieved in busy radiology practices (though becoming much more common in the PACS environment). Extraneous light coming from the view box around the film decreases the sensitivity of the eye for detecting subtle changes in contrast in the denser portion of the image (again, virtually eliminated with PACS). Although faulty search patterns and radiologist carelessness may sometimes be responsible for errors, the major limitations in the detection of lung nodules are inherent to the human visual system, the complexity of the underlying anatomy, the plain film method itself, or the location and edge characteristics of the tumor itself.[34] Therefore, the failure to detect an early lung cancer on plain radiographs is well within an accepted standard of care and does not necessarily constitute negligence or malpractice.[35]

Inadequate Exposure or Positioning[36]

The accuracy of a radiologist can be no greater than the quality of the radiographs presented for interpretation. Although technologists may physically perform the examinations, the radiologist who interprets them has the ultimate legal responsibility for a technically inadequate radiograph that fails to show an abnormality.

All radiologic facilities should have written policies that describe the imaging views required and the technical factors to be used for all radiographic examinations. Nevertheless, technique charts or routine phototimer settings may not always result in ideally exposed radiographs. Consequently, it is up to radiologists to use their best judgment to determine whether a radiograph can be properly interpreted if it is overexposed (with the use of a bright light), underexposed, or poorly positioned. If a study is readable but not ideal, radiologists should document the technical limitations in the formal dictation, adding that it nevertheless is still of "reasonable diagnostic quality." This contemporaneous record enables radiologists to explain and even defend their judgment in the future, if the case becomes the subject of a malpractice suit.

If a radiologist is convinced that a study cannot be properly interpreted because of inadequate exposure or positioning, an immediate repeat radiograph should be obtained if the patient is still available. If the patient has already left the department, the radiologist should make a formal dictation indicating that the study cannot be interpreted, giving the reasons why and indicating that repeat radiographs have been requested. The radiologist should attempt to recall the patient directly and, if this is not possible, should contact the referring physician with a request to do so. In either scenario, the radiologist should document the recall or attempted recall in the report.

At times, the physical condition of the patient may prevent the technologist from completing an examination with all required views or with optimal exposure techniques. If this makes it impossible to properly interpret the study, the radiologist should clearly state in the report that the examination was incomplete because of the patient's condition. The report should specify which views were not obtained or what anatomic areas were not sufficiently visualized, and then recommend that repeat or follow-up views should be obtained when the patient's condition permits.

Meticulous and careful positioning is especially critical in the patient who has sustained cervical spine trauma. Missing a fracture or dislocation in the cervical region can lead to huge malpractice awards due to the high financial costs of caring for a patient who is quadriplegic, particularly one who is young and has a long life expectancy. Consequently, each radiology facility should have a written policy that specifies the additional views (swimmer's, obliques) or imaging procedures (computed tomography) to be performed if the routine cross-table lateral view fails to adequately visualize the lower cervical spine and cervicothoracic junction in a patient with neck trauma. If the patient's condition precludes the technologist from obtaining such views or additional studies, this information should be verbally communicated to the referring physician, along with a request that a repeat examination be obtained when the patient's condition permits. The inability to complete the study, and any contact with the referring physician, should be documented in the formal report.

Admitting Errors

What should radiologists say after making errors? This is a critical ethical and legal issue that may have a substantial effect on both the likelihood of becoming subjected to a malpractice lawsuit and the eventual result of any litigation.

All radiologists agree that, "because of ethical, medical, and legal considerations, radiologists should promptly and completely divulge to patients or patients' families the occurrence and nature of any complication or adverse event that takes place during a diagnostic or therapeutic radiologic procedure."[37] Although one may be tempted to cover up the fact that an error has taken place, this probably constitutes ineffective or even counterproductive risk management. Because modern medical care tends to be "a complex enterprise involving so many different professionals potentially interacting with the patient, the medical chart, and external evaluators (including attorneys), [from a pragmatic point of view] it is unlikely that a cover-up of essential facts about a medical error relating to serious patient harm could be sustained indefinitely." Moreover, studies have shown that "the majority of patients and surrogates expect, respect, and reward honesty" on the part of their physicians.[38] One article[39] reported that virtually all patients want their physicians to offer some kind of acknowledgment or apology for even minor errors. Contrary to general perception, the failure to disclose mistakes may almost double the risk of a patient's pursuing a malpractice suit and substantially increase the likelihood of a complaint's being filed with a state medical board. Another study of the families of neonates suffering complications[40] found that 24% of those who sued did so because of a perception that the physician had not been completely honest about the cause of an adverse event, and almost half of these families resented that their doctors had misled them.

When discussing a complication, radiologists should honestly describe what happened in an objective and factual manner, avoiding "doubletalk" meant merely to confound the issue. However, there is significant disagreement about whether there is an obligation to "disclose whether, and the degree to which, the complication may have been caused by a radiologist's mistake or error."[41]

According to ivory-tower ethicists, physicians are obliged to immediately and completely admit to patients any mistakes made while per-

forming diagnostic or therapeutic procedures.[42,43] However, this is not
the practice in real life. In a study of house officers in internal medicine,[44] less than one quarter of those who had made serious medical
mistakes actually informed the affected patients or their families about
them. This and a subsequent study[45] of practicing physicians revealed
multiple reasons for reluctance to admit mistakes—guilt or shame; fear
of being criticized or ostracized by peers and supervisors; potential economic consequences such as loss of referrals, hospital admitting privileges, or preferred provider status; and the possible revocation of medical
licensure. Nevertheless, by far the major reason is probably the fear
that such a confession would provoke a medical malpractice suit.

It is essential to distinguish between admitting the fact that something has gone wrong and volunteering the opinion that oneself or another member of the health care team was negligent. "Not all mistakes
fall to the level of a deviation from professionally acceptable standards
of care." Therefore, "the physician's obligation to be truthful extends
only to acknowledging that a mistake happened, not to personally con-
ceding or accusing others of legal fault."[46]

Insurers and medical-legal experts faced with the practicality of increasing
malpractice lawsuits vehemently argue that physicians should not admit to
making medical errors. According to a representative of a major insurance
company, urging doctors to confess their mistakes is "asking them to commit professional suicide."[47] As another expert observed, "If you tell the
truth, apologize and reach out to a family in grief, you can diffuse some of
the anger ... but every word you utter is an admission that can be used
against you in a court of law."[48] These warnings are well founded, for
extrajudicial (out-of-court) admissions can be devastating at a subsequent
trial. When a plaintiff cannot provide independent expert testimony to support a claim, the defense will move for the judge to grant a summary judgment dismissing the case. However, as one appellate court ruled, "It is a
generally accepted proposition that the necessary expert testimony [to show
that the physician was negligent] may consist of admissions by the defendant doctor."[49] In many cases, extrajudicial statements made by a physician to a patient or patient's family outside of the courtroom may be
admissible in evidence at trial. "The defendant-physician can either refute
the alleged admission or at least offer information to mitigate its importance. The jury is then left to decide how much weight, if any, to give these
statements in their deliberation to determine whether the physician-defen-
dant breached the standard of care."[50]

How should radiologists handle the situation? When initially speaking
with patients, radiologists should be compassionate and caring for the
patient's plight. Although it is appropriate to express sorrow for what
has happened, words such as "apologize" should be avoided lest the

patient consider them as an admission of physician error. Radiologists should not speculate about the cause of a complication and never cast blame on others or themselves. Phrases such as "It is my fault," "I messed/goofed up," or "I am to blame for this" should never be used since they are tantamount to an admission of negligence or carelessness that can come back to haunt a radiologist later at trial. "If it is not immediately known whether the complication is the result of an error, the radiologist should inform the patient that an investigation will be conducted to determine the cause of the complication, and [that] the patient will be apprised of the findings."[51]

There is some disagreement as to what radiologists should say if they sincerely believe that they have made a mistake that resulted in an injury to the patient. Berlin argues that radiologists are "ethically and professionally bound to divulge this fact to the patient … [in] phrases such as 'I believe I have made an error,' or 'This complication may be due to an inadvertent error on my part'.… [This] conveys to the patient a truthful representation of what may have happened, but with less likelihood of legal self-incrimination.'"[52] Others, taking a sober view of the current litigious nature of society, would strongly disagree. Most malpractice insurance policies instruct physicians not to admit fault to patients, regardless of the words in which it is phrased. As the legal counsel of a national professional liability insurance company noted, "If you have a doctor out there saying, 'Oh, I did it,' it's a little hard for those of us who write the insurance."[53] Other consultants echo that theme, instructing physicians to show humility if they have made a mistake but to never indicate or imply in any way that they were negligent or careless.[54]

Reporting the "Missed" Diagnosis

All too frequently, the radiologist is faced with the ethical and medicolegal dilemma of how to handle the situation in which a radiologic image, previously reported as normal, in retrospect reveals a malignancy. Should radiologists include in their reports (and inform the referring physician) that a presumably malignant lesion on the current study was actually present but missed on a previous examination, or should they not mention the original images and only report on the current ones?[55]

There are numerous reasons for remaining silent in the face of a previously missed lesion. Directly stating in a radiology report that a malignancy was overlooked is a veritable "red flag" or "smoking gun" to a malpractice attorney. This is especially important in cases in which there are no other medical grounds in the patient's chart on which to file a negligence action. In addition, any person with access to the report (secretaries, clerks, medical record librarians, nurses) may decide to pass this information along to an attorney in exchange for a "finder's fee."[56] Reporting the missed finding of a colleague could label a radiologist as a "fink" who "squealed" on a partner, and such conduct virtually guarantees that the radiologist will be called to testify if the case ever goes to trial. Reporting one's own missed finding is ethically admirable, but may well be an open invitation to a malpractice lawsuit.

The American College of Radiology has not published any standards regarding whether a radiologist has a professional obligation to document a previously missed diagnosis. However, there is a standard requiring radiologists to compare current studies with previous radiologic examinations "when appropriate and available," so that failure to mention the missed diagnosis in a report would be a technical violation.[57] Similarly, the Code of Medical Ethics of the American Medical Association is silent concerning whether a physician has an obligation to inform a patient that an error has been committed.[58]

As Berlin has written, "the preponderance of legal opinion, as enunciated in various state appellate courts, favors complete disclosure by the physician of all facts and information relevant to a patient's health or well-being, including complications of medical procedures and iatrogenic errors and injuries."[59] This is related to the fiduciary obligation to disclose everything that is in the best interest of the patient, so that the patient can make an intelligent decision regarding treatment.[60] However, the radiologist has no legal duty to disclose to the patient an error or a missed radiologic diagnosis, just as physicians are not required to disclose an act of malpractice to either the patient or to another third party.[61] Although a missed diagnosis of malignancy is unquestionably an "adverse event," whether it is sufficient to constitute negligence is a legal decision to be made by a finder of fact (judge or jury) and not within the purview of an individual physician.[62]

Nevertheless, the radiologist who chooses not to report an overlooked abnormality should be aware of possible (even if unlikely) legal consequences of this action. One is a charge of *fraudulent concealment*—the failure to disclose material facts when one should do so. The physician may be deemed to have violated the law if it can be proven that he or she "*intended* to conceal an act of negligence by destroying, altering, or hiding relevant reports or radiologic images ... [or deliberately] provided misinformation that prevented the patient from obtaining the true facts."[63] However, for a physician to be liable the fraud must be of "such character as to prevent inquiry, elude investigation, or mislead the patient" who has undertaken "due diligence" to discover the specific medical information that was allegedly concealed.[64] As long as the films on which the lesion was present but missed are not sequestered and are available for review by an independent radiologist retained by the plaintiff's attorney, the legal criteria for a charge of fraudulent concealment appear to be absent.[65] Furthermore, courts have ruled that simply withholding information that is based on "speculation, conjecture, or mere possibility" is not sufficient to make a physician liable for fraudulent concealment; rather, the physician must have failed to reveal medical information on errors that he or she knows to be at least "probable."[66] This would appear to permit a radiologist to avoid disclosing an apparent error when its detection may have been difficult to discover on the initial examination. Furthermore, disclosure of information that would be of no value for current patient treatment but would be used solely for the purpose of a malpractice lawsuit would appear not to be required in view of a judicial decision indicating that a physician does not have to disclose information material to a patient's *nonmedical* interests or rights (such as something that may influence a patient's business or investment affairs).[67]

Radiologists who decide to report a previous misdiagnosis should do so in a matter-of-fact, nonjudgmental manner. Berlin recommends a statement such as: "In retrospect, the lesion was present on the radiograph of ..." Under no circumstances should one employ such words as "error" or "mistake"; potentially inflammatory phrases such as "should have been diagnosed" or "was obviously present but not seen" should be avoided.[68]

Whether or not to disclose a previously missed diagnosis is ultimately the choice of the individual radiologist, who must weigh the value of ethical purity and complete compliance with professional standards against the possibility of being the catalyst that precipitates a malpractice lawsuit.

Defending the "Missed" Radiographic Diagnosis

"Once an abnormality shown on a radiograph is pointed out and becomes so obvious that laypersons such as judges, juries, and other attorneys can see it, it is not easy to convince anyone that a radiologist who is trained and paid for seeing the lesion should be exonerated for missing it. No wonder most of these cases are settled before trial with payment to the patient."[69] Nevertheless, there are arguments that can be raised by a skilled attorney that may be sufficiently persuasive that they result in a trial verdict in favor of the defendant radiologist.[70]

The most powerful judicial ruling in the arsenal of the attorney representing a defendant radiologist is the 1997 opinion of the Wisconsin Court of Appeals[71] confirming a circuit court ruling[72] that directly addressed the issue of perceptual errors. It stressed that medicine is "not an exact science, and even the best of physicians can be wrong in diagnosis or procedure. The question, however, is not whether a physician has made a mistake; rather, the question is whether he was negligent. Unless the untoward result was caused by the failure to conform to the accepted standard of care, he is not liable on negligence." The circuit court observed that the term "reasonable physician" is preferable to "average physician," because those with less than "average" skill may still be competent and qualified. "Half of the physicians of America do not automatically become negligent in practicing medicine … merely because their skills are less than the professional average." Thus, failure of a defendant-radiologist to detect what an "average" radiologist should have detected is not *ipso facto* negligence. Rather, "negligence is determined by whether the defendant radiologist failed to use reasonable and ordinary care." Radiologists "simply cannot detect all abnormalities on all x-rays." As the circuit court concluded, all radiologists should be expected to see "obvious" lesions but may not see those that are "subtle." To expect all radiologists to see every subtle lesion would be "to elevate the average physician to the perfect physician, and perfection is a standard to which no profession can possibly adhere." Thus, "Errors in perception by radiologists viewing x-rays occur in the absence of negligence."

Defense attorneys can call expert witnesses to testify to statistics regarding the "frequency of errors committed by radiologists and other physicians during the course of daily practice; the factors that cause varying conspicuity of radiographic densities; the limitations of normal human visual perception"; the subtlety of the lesion in question; and evidence that the conduct of the defendant-radiologist was careful and prudent.[73] Another approach is a defense based on an analogy between the missed lesion on a radiograph and the illustrations in the *Where's Waldo?* books written by Martin Handford.[74] In these illustrations, it initially is extremely difficult to find Waldo hidden among the many other faces in a picture. Once found or pointed out, however, Waldo becomes obvious and easily detected the next time one views it. Similarly, it can be argued that it is a difficult task to find an abnormal shadow among the multitude of shadows of varying density on a radiograph, whereas both Waldo and a radiographic abnormality can be seen quickly and clearly in retrospect.[75] By extension, therefore, the conduct of a radiologist should be judged according to the process by which he or she initially interpreted the radiograph, rather than the accuracy of the interpretation itself.[76]

In addition, defense attorneys can argue that retrospective viewing of images by an expert witness retained by the plaintiff bears little relationship to the situation of the defendant when rendering the initial interpretation. "The retrospective reader frequently has access to information regarding the patient's subsequent course, including later radiographs demonstrating more advanced disease ... [which] substantially improves the observer's ability to perceive subtle abnormalities.... Perception is better if you know where to look and what to look for." The visual information sufficient for radiologic diagnosis may not actually be present on an earlier radiograph, but only in the relation between earlier and later studies. Therefore, the "retrospectoscope" should not be considered an accurate reflection of radiologic reality.[77]

Of course, none of these various defensive strategies may prove successful. Nevertheless, they at least offer some hope in defending the "missed" radiographic diagnosis.

Endnotes

1 Kohn LT, Corrigan JM, Donaldson MS, eds. To Err Is Human: Building a Safer Health System. Washington, DC: National Academy, 1999.

2 McDonald CJ, Weiner M, Hui SL. Deaths due to medical errors are exaggerated in Institute of Medicine report. *JAMA* 2000;284:93–95.

3 Brennan TA, Leape LL, Laird NM, et al. Incidence of adverse events and negligence in hospitalized patients: results of the Harvard medical practice study. *N Engl J Med* 1991;324:370–376.

4 Thomas EJ, Studdert DM, Burstin HR, et al. Incidence and types of adverse events and negligent care in Utah and Colorado. *Med Care* 2000;38:261–271.

5 Garland LH. On the scientific evaluation of diagnostic procedures. *Radiology* 1949;52:309–328.

6 Berlin L. The missed breast cancer: perceptions and realities. *AJR* 1999;173:1161–1167.

7 Muhm JR, Miller WE, Fontana RS, et al. Lung cancer detected during a screening program using four-month chest radiographs. *Radiology* 1983;148:609–615.

8 Berlin L. Defending the "missed" radiographic diagnosis. *AJR* 2001;176:317–322.

9 Siegle RL, Baram EM, Reuter SR, et al. Rates of disagreement in imaging interpretation in a group of community hospitals. *Acad Radiol* 1998;5:148–154.

10 Brennan TA, Leape LL, Laird NM, et al. Incidence of adverse events and negligence in hospitalized patients: results of the Harvard medical practice study. *N Engl J Med* 1991;324:370–376.

11 Thomas EJ, Studdert DM, Burstin HR, et al. Incidence and types of adverse events and negligent care in Utah and Colorado. *Med Care* 2000;38:261–271.

12 Yerushalmy J. The statistical assessment of variability in observer perception and description of roentgenographic pulmonary shadows. *Radiol Clin North Am* 1969;7:381–392.

13 Berlin L. Perceptual errors. *AJR* 1996;157:587–590.

14 Berlin L, Hendrix RW. Perceptual errors and negligence. *AJR* 1998;170:863–867.

15 Berlin L. Perceptual errors. *AJR* 1996;157:587–590.

16 Berlin L. Possessing ordinary knowledge. *AJR* 1996;166:1027–1029.

17 Ibid.

18 Berlin L. Errors in judgment. *AJR* 1996;166:1259–1261.

19 *Spike v Sellett*, 102 Ill App 3d 270, 430 NE2d 597 (1981).

20 Brennan TA, Hebert LE, Laird N, et al. Hospital characteristics associated with adverse events and substandard care. *JAMA* 1991;265:3265–3269.

21 *Riggins v Mauriello*, 603 A2d 827 (Del 1992).

22 Berlin L. Errors in judgment. *AJR* 1996;166:1259–1261.

23 Berlin L, Hendrix RW. Perceptual errors and negligence. *AJR* 1998;170:863–867.

24 Potchen EJ, Bisesi MA. When is it malpractice to miss lung cancer on chest radiographs? *Radiology* 1990;175:29–32.

25 Berlin L, Hendrix RW. Perceptual errors and negligence. *AJR* 1998;170:863–867.

26 Berbaum KS, El-Khoury GY, Franken EA Jr, et al. Impact of clinical history on fracture detection with radiography. *Radiology* 1988;168:507–511.

27 Ibid.

28 Berbaum KS, Franken EA Jr, El-Khoury GY. Impact of clinical history on radiographic detection of fractures: a comparison of radiologists and orthopedists. *AJR* 1989;153:1221–1224.

29 Woodring JH. Pitfalls in the radiologic diagnosis of lung cancer. *AJR* 1990;154:1165–1175.

30 Kundel HL, Nodine CF, Thickman D, Toto L. Searching for lung nodules: a comparison of human performance with random and systematic scanning models. *Invest Radiol* 1987;22:417–422.

31 Oestmann JW, Greene R, Kushner DC, et al. Lung lesions: correlation between viewing time and detection. *Radiology* 1988;166:451–453.

32 Kundel HL, Nodine CF, Thickman D, Toto L. Searching for lung nodules: a comparison of human performance with random and systematic scanning models. *Invest Radiol* 1987;22:417–422.

33 Jaffe CC. Medical imaging, vision, and visual psychophysics. *Med Radiogr Photogr* 1984;60:1–48.

34 Woodring JH. Pitfalls in the radiologic diagnosis of lung cancer. *AJR* 1990;154:1165–1175.

35 Muhm JR, Miller WE, Fontana RS, et al. Lung cancer detected during a screening program using four-month chest radiographs. *Radiology* 1983;148:609–615.

36 Berlin L. The importance of proper radiographic positioning and technique. *AJR* 1996;166:769–771.
37 Berlin L. Reporting the "missed" radiologic diagnosis: medicolegal and ethical considerations. *Radiology* 1994;192:183–187.
38 Kapp MB. Medical mistakes and older patients: admitting errors and improving care. *J Am Geriatr Soc* 2001;45:1361–1365.
39 Witman AB, Park DM, Hardin SE. How do patients want physicians to handle mistakes? *Arch Intern Med* 1996;156:2565–2569.
40 Hickson GB, Wright Clayton E, Githens PB, Sloan FA. Factors that prompted families to file medical malpractice claims following perinatal injuries. *JAMA* 1992;267:1359015–1363.
41 Berlin L. Admitting mistakes. *AJR* 1999;172:879–884.
42 Applegate WB. Physician management of patients with adverse outcomes. *Arch Intern Med* 1986;146:2249–2252.
43 Witman AB, Park DM, Hardin SE. How do patients want physicians to handle mistakes? *Arch Intern Med* 1996;156:2565–2569.
44 Wu AW, Folkman S, McPhee SJ, Lo B. Do house officers learn from their mistakes? *JAMA* 1991;265:2089–2094.
45 Wu AW, Cavanaugh TA, McPhee SJ, et al. To tell the truth: ethical and practical issues in disclosing medical mistakes to patients. *J Gen Intern Med* 1997;12:770–775.
46 Kapp MB. Medical mistakes and older patients: admitting errors and improving care. *J Am Geriatr Soc* 2001;45:1361–1365.
47 Grady D. Doctors urged to admit mistakes. New York Times, December 9, 1997:B15.
48 Ibid.
49 *Jarboe v Harting*, 397 SW2d 775 (Ky App 1965).
50 Berlin L. Admitting mistakes. *AJR* 1999;172:879–884.
51 Ibid.
52 Ibid.
53 Grady D. Doctors urged to admit mistakes. New York Times, December 9, 1997:B15.
54 Tennenhouse DJ, Kasher MP. *Risk Prevention Skills: Communicating and Record Keeping in Clinical Practice*. Corte Madera, CA: Tennenhouse Professional Publications, 1995:109–113,121–127.
55 Berlin L. Reporting the "missed" radiologic diagnosis: medicolegal and ethical considerations. *AJR* 1994;192:183–187.
56 Ibid.
57 *ACR Standard for Communication: Diagnostic Radiology*. Reston, VA: American College of Radiology, 2000–2001.
58 Berlin L. Reporting the "missed" radiologic diagnosis: medicolegal and ethical considerations. *AJR* 1994;192:183–187.
59 Ibid.
60 Rhodes M. Duties of physicians. In: Zaremski M, Goldstein LS, eds. *Hospital and Medical Negligence*. Deerfield, IL: Callaghan, 1988:50–53.

61 Vogel J, Delgado R. To tell the truth: the physician's duty to disclose medical mistakes. *UCLA Law Rev* 1980;28:52–94.

62 Berlin L. Reporting the "missed" radiologic diagnosis: medicolegal and ethical considerations. *AJR* 1994;192:183–187.

63 Ibid.

64 *Muller v Thaut*, 230 Neb 244, 430 NW2d 884 (Neb 1988).

65 Berlin L. Reporting the "missed" radiologic diagnosis: medicolegal and ethical considerations. *AJR* 1994;192:183–187.

66 *Valdez v Lyman-Roberts Hospital, Inc*, 638 SW2d 111 (Tex App 1982).

67 *Arato v Avedon*, 5 Cal 4th 1172, 858 P2d 598, 23 Cal Rptr 2d 131 (Calif 1993).

68 Berlin L. Reporting the "missed" radiologic diagnosis: medicolegal and ethical considerations. *AJR* 1994;192:183–187.

69 Berlin L. Perceptual errors. *AJR* 1996;157:587–590.

70 Berlin L. Defending the "missed" radiographic diagnosis. *AJR* 2001; 176:317–322.

71 *Department of Regulation and Licensing v State of Wisconsin Medical Examining Board*, 572 NW2d 505 (Wis App 1997).

72 *State of Wisconsin Department of Regulation and Licensing v State of Wisconsin Medical Examining Board and George E. Farley, MD*. 96-CV-0657 (Dane County, Wis 1996).

73 Berlin L, Hendrix RW. Perceptual errors and negligence. *AJR* 1998;170: 863–867.

74 Handford M. *Where's Waldo?* Boston: Little, Brown, 1987.

75 Hendrix RW. In defense of a missed lesion (letter). *Radiology* 1995;195: 578.

76 Berlin L, Hendrix RW. Perceptual errors and negligence. *AJR* 1998;170: 863–867.

77 Berbaum KS. Difficulty of judging retrospectively whether a diagnosis has been "missed" (letter). *Radiology* 1995;194:582–583.

15
Interpreting Too Many Studies Per Day

Can a radiologist be held liable for missing a lesion because he or she was "overworked" by interpreting too many studies in one day? This rare allegation may become more popular among plaintiffs' attorneys because of the current combination of a shortage of radiologists and an increasing number of imaging examinations.

The seminal study on radiology workload revealed that radiologists in a group practice interpreted an average of about 11,000 imaging procedures per year.[1] The authors stressed that their workload data showed substantial variability, citing another study in which the average annual workload ranged up to 17,900 studies. The article contained a disclaimer emphasizing that average yearly workloads are influenced by many factors, including the type of radiologic procedure and complexity of the findings; whether previous studies were available for comparison; whether it was the radiologist or some other personnel who hung the radiographs on the view box or alternator; whether the radiologist was constantly being interrupted by telephone or in-person consultations with referring physicians; whether the radiologist had additional administrative, research, or teaching duties; the varying speeds at which different radiologists work; and the number of hours the radiologist worked in a given day. The increasing utilization of PACS technology should also affect average productivity statistics. Although this and subsequent articles urged that their results not in any way be considered to reflect the standard of care, the raw data in workload studies are potentially dangerous for practicing radiologists who are efficient, work long hours, and can devote their entire day to interpreting imaging examinations.

Assuming that the average radiologist works about 250 days a year, the average workload per radiologist ranges from 50 to 70 diagnostic procedures per day.[2] This would be extremely high (if not impossible) for a radiologist reading only CT or MRI scans, but far too low for one interpreting only plain films. For those interpreting mammograms, a major textbook states that most radiologists can interpret 40 to 50 studies in a 2-hour session, as long as the current and previous films are placed on an alternator so that film handling by the radiologist is minimized.[3] A Swedish study reported an average workload per radiologist of 150 to 200 screening mammograms per day.[4]

Several articles have evaluated the question of how much time a radiologist must devote to interpret accurately an individual imaging examination. Ironically, in one study radiologists averaged more time interpreting those cases in which errors were made than they spent on the examinations diagnosed correctly![5] A subsequent article[6] reported that a large number of true-positive observations were made during the first few seconds of search. By comparing radiographs with a previously learned concept of normal, radiologists detected obvious abnormalities almost immediately, with the number of abnormalities detected increasing with the experience of the observer. Nevertheless, longer searches did result in an increased number of positive observations. Even though the authors recognized that the value of a long search time in interpreting images is overestimated, the article concluded that the radiologist who interprets an examination in a few seconds is gambling that a large proportion of radiographs show normal findings.[7] Another study, however, has cautioned that a quarter of subtle lung lesions are missed even with unlimited viewing time.[8] Moreover, longer viewing times are associated with an increased incidence of false positives, resulting in workups for lesions that do not exist.

Despite multiple studies, there are no scientific data to set workload numbers or interpretation times that could constitute a legally valid standard of care. Nevertheless, since enterprising plaintiffs' attorneys may cite specific studies as evidence to support their claims of negligence related to overwork and fatigue, radiologists should consider methods to thwart this attempt. As Berlin has noted,[9] as a useful deterrent to unfounded allegations, radiology groups should consider including in their group or department policy a reference to workload parameters, such as: "The daily workload for radiologists in the group is variable, depending on their specific duties and the degree of staffing for the department." If a portion of the remuneration of radiologists is related to individual productivity, the group should stress in a policy statement that "productivity is a far less important factor in the determination of income than the providing of optimal patient care, which is the group's primary goal." Radiologists must make certain that the attention and care they devote to the last examination of the day is as intense as that for the first imaging study. Radiologists who feel "fatigued or not able to devote their full energy toward interpreting a radiologic study should either delay the interpretation until they are adequately rested or ask a radiology colleague to provide the interpretation instead."

Endnotes

1 Sunshine JH, Bansal MS. Operational characteristics of radiology groups in the United States in 1992. *Radiology* 1994;193:613–618.

2 Berlin L. Liability of interpreting too many radiographs. *AJR* 2000;175:17–22.

3 Kopans DB. *Breast Imaging, 2nd ed.* Philadelphia: Lippincott-Raven 1998: 211–212.

4 Thurfjell EL, Lernevall KA, Taube AAS. Benefit of independent double reading in a population-based screening program. *Radiology* 1994;191: 241–244.

5 Lehr JL, Lodwick GS, Farrell C, et al. Direct measurement of the effect of film miniaturization on diagnostic accuracy. *Radiology* 1976;118:257–263.

6 Christensen EE, Murray RC, Holland K, et al. The effect of search time on perception. *Radiology* 1981;138:361–365.

7 Berlin L. Liability of interpreting too many radiographs. *AJR* 2000;175: 17–22.

8 Oestmann JW, Greene R, Kushner DC, et al. Lung lesions: correlation between viewing time and detection. *Radiology* 1988;166:451–453.

9 Berlin L. Liability of interpreting too many radiographs. *AJR* 2000;175: 17–22.

Part III
Communication and Records

16
Radiology Reports

Written interpretations by radiologists of imaging studies are extremely important from both the medical and legal perspectives. They are an integral part of the medical record and an essential link between the diagnosis and treatment of a patient's illness.[1] The radiology report should accurately and concisely describe the positive imaging findings and any relevant negative findings, as well as provide an opinion as to their significance.[2] If there is a specific clinical question presented in the request form, the report should attempt to answer it clearly and directly. Whenever possible, there should be a differential diagnosis with relative probabilities. As the American College of Radiology (ACR) Standard for Communication[3] notes, when appropriate the radiology report should contain an impression including "a precise diagnosis" and a recommendation for "follow-up or additional diagnostic studies to clarify or confirm the impression." A rambling description of findings without a reasonable conclusion may only leave the reader confused.[4] The length of the body of the report depends on the number of findings, whereas the length of the conclusion reflects the ability of the radiologist to make sense of the findings.[5]

The radiology report should clearly convey to the referring physician three critical items: (a) the imaging findings; (b) the underlying pathologic process (limited differential diagnosis or the precise etiology); and (c) recommendations for further studies or clinical investigation. Although often considered the trademark (or official shrub) of the profession, radiologists should avoid the "hedge"—"the making of calculatedly noncommittal or ambiguous statements."[6] If the radiologist believes that a lesion may be malignant, he or she should clearly state that it is "suspicious for cancer" rather than confusing the issue with vague and meaningless phraseology. In malpractice actions for the delayed diagnosis of malignancy, referring physicians frequently (and often successfully) attempt to shift the blame to the radiologist for not issuing a strong enough report that would have caused them to pursue the proper diagnosis sooner.

A controversial issue is whether referring clinicians prefer radiology reports to be short or detailed and whether reports should include recommendations for further studies. Although one Canadian study[7] reported that 95% of clinicians wanted radiology reports to include such recommendations, another[8] noted that this was desired by more than half of general practitioners but only one third of internists and surgeons. General practitioners also preferred long lists of differential diagnoses, unlike surgeons who "appreciated brevity with telegraphic style." Similar differences were observed in an American study,[9] which found that "many referring physicians value the radiologist as a lesion detector more than as a lesion interpreter … [trusting] in their own abilities to determine what it means." This view especially applied to specialists, such as orthopedists and neurosurgeons, rather than generalists. Some complained that "radiologists recommend too many additional imaging studies that are not really indicated, yet must be performed for medicolegal reasons, once mentioned in the radiology report."

According to the ACR Standards for Communication,[10] when appropriate the radiologist should unequivocally recommend an additional imaging study or biopsy, rather than employ such terms as "if clinically warranted" or "if clinically indicated." Similarly, radiologists should avoid such vague phrases as "comparison with previous films may be of benefit" or "clinical correlation is recommended" when assessing abnormal radiographic findings. As Berlin has observed,[11] "Because radiologists are acknowledged to possess radiologic expertise derived from training and experience, they should not relinquish to nonradiology physicians the responsibility of evaluating the potential significance of a purely radiographic finding that is unexpected or unusual."

Ironically, specialists who do not wish to have radiologists include in their reports recommendations for additional studies often have a dramatic change of opinion when these same physicians are named as defendants in a medical malpractice lawsuit. All of a sudden, these nonradiologist physicians typically claim that they relied heavily on the radiology report and would have ordered additional imaging studies if only they had been suggested. Indeed, the degree of reliance on the radiologist may be a key factor in determining how courts assess the comparative liability of various medical codefendants.[12]

Most radiologists provide a detailed description of the imaging findings in the body of the report, followed by a concise impression or conclusion. This enables the referring physician to easily see the radiologist's final opinion without necessarily having to wade through the observations and thought processes that led up to it. The use of clinically supplied information within the radiology report remains a subject of debate. "Some recommend that it be included at the beginning of each report, others suggest that it be incorporated in the body of the report, still others suggest that it should be used in the conclusion, and finally some claim that it should not be used at all."[13]

The final report should be checked carefully to correct any typographical errors and to detect any possible inconsistencies (e.g., right and left) before it is signed. It is especially critical to make certain that the words *no* and *not* were not inadvertently skipped by the transcriptionist, an omission that completely changes the interpretation. Radiologists should always be aware that a properly worded report can be a deciding factor in the successful defense of a malpractice lawsuit. A correct diagnosis that is improperly stated (or incorrectly or inadequately transmitted to the referring physician) can be catastrophic at trial.[14]

Comparison with Previous Examinations and Reports[15]

It is a generally accepted principle in the radiology and legal communities that radiologists have a duty to compare current radiographs with previous studies.[16] Therefore, it is essential that a system be in place so that the radiologist knows whether the patient has had prior examinations at that facility.

The radiology report should always mention that the examination has been compared with one or more previous studies. If the patient has not been seen before in the department, it is prudent for the radiologist to state that fact in the report, even if the radiologist has no reason to believe that comparison with previous films is necessary in this particular case.

Previous radiographs from the facility may be unavailable for a variety of reasons, such as their being in remote storage or having been lost or checked out to a third party. If they will not be easily accessible, the radiologist may render a report based on the current radiographs, noting that the previous studies were unavailable. If the radiologist believes that reviewing the previous films would aid in making an appropriate interpretation of the current study, it would be prudent to add that he or she will issue a follow-up report including a comparison with the prior examination once it is made available. Although the decision to keep old radiographs in remote storage is usually a policy determined by the hospital because of space limitations, the radiologist has an independent duty to make a good-faith effort to retrieve previous films and compare them with the current study.

The radiologist should indicate in the formal written report whether a comparison with previous studies obtained at another facility would be vital for proper evaluation of the current examination. In such cases, courts have ruled that the radiologist must make a good-faith effort to obtain these previous films by notifying the referring physician, the patient, or both, indicating that a new and more complete report will be issued once the prior study is available and a comparison has been made.

Radiologists generally compare the current radiographic examination with the most recent previous study. Exceptions include the need to review chest radiographs dating back at least two years to determine that an unchanging pulmonary nodule most likely represents a benign granuloma, and that an unchanging apical process is most consistent with old tuberculosis rather than an active lesion. In one malpractice suit, the jury decided that the defendant radiologist had a duty to review all previously obtained radiographs,[17] though this is probably an aberration and obviously impractical in a busy hospital setting.

When prior films for comparison are not immediately available, radiologists often are content to read the previous radiology reports. However, this can be a dangerous practice, for there is no assurance that the previous examinations were interpreted correctly! If the radiologist deems that comparison with prior studies is truly necessary for proper analysis of the current examination, it is far safer to either withhold a formal report until viewing the old films or to offer to render an amended report once they are available.

Significant Discrepancy Between the Final and Emergency/Preliminary Reports

Any significant discrepancy between an emergency or preliminary report and the final written report should be promptly reconciled by direct communication between the radiologist and the referring physician, other health care provider, or an appropriate representative. When radiographs are interpreted by emergency room physicians because no radiologist is on the premises (either in small hospitals or after normal hours in larger institutions without on-call residents), a system should be established by which the non-radiologist indicates an interpretation for each examination. A radiologist detecting any significant differences when viewing the studies the next day must immediately telephone the emergency department (or, if possible, preferably bring the radiographs to the emergency room), so that the patient is promptly brought back for appropriate care. This action should always be documented in the formal report. Failure to notify the emergency department of the error in an expeditious fashion can expose the radiologist to substantial legal liability.

Signing the Radiology Report[18]

As an integral part of the patient's medical record, the radiology report must accurately reflect the radiologist's interpretation. However, many radiologists treat their reports in a cavalier fashion, signing all of them at the end of the day without reading them carefully or even verifying that they actually had interpreted them. The ACR Standard for Communication: Diagnostic Radiology (2000) states, "The final report should be proofread to minimize typographical errors, deleted words, and confusing or conflicting statements." Electronic or rubber-stamp signature devices, instead of a written signature, are acceptable as long as access to them is secure.

The Health Care Financing Administration (HCFA) currently requires that "the radiologist or other practitioner who performs radiology services must sign reports of his or her interpretations." In contrast, the Joint Commission on Accreditation of Healthcare Organizations (JCAHO) mandates only that "every medical record entry is dated, its author identified, and, when necessary, authenticated [to verify that an entry is complete, accurate, and final]." By including the phrase "when necessary, authenticated," JCAHO has effectively eliminated its blanket requirement that all radiology reports must be reviewed and signed by the radiologist who rendered the service, instead giving each hospital the discretion to decide whether signatures are needed in all cases.

Although in practice radiologists sign virtually all reports, few can honestly state that they unequivocally convey the meaning that was intended. It is difficult, if not impossible, for radiologists to verify the accuracy of every report based on an interpretation rendered many hours (or even days) earlier, at the time the radiologic study was performed. Serious transcription errors, such as confusing left with right or inserting or deleting the words "no" or "not," can easily occur and would probably not be noted by a radiologist signing a large number of reports at one time. Realistically, eliminating this ever-present potential source of error must await the dissemination of voice-recognition technology, which immediately generates a report that the radiologist can authenticate at the time.

Referring physicians and third-party payers alike demand rapid turnaround time for radiology reports. This presents a significant problem for radiology practices, whose members generate a large number of reports daily yet take time off for illness, vacation, and attending continuing medical education courses. Nevertheless, radiologists are frequently requested, or even compelled, to sign reports for colleagues who are unable to do so in a timely manner. In virtually every case, the radiologist who signs a colleague's report does not review the images on which the transcribed dictation was based and, therefore, may finalize a report that contains inaccurate or erroneous information. Of course, the interpreting radiologist will have legal exposure for any errors contained in the final written report, even if that radiologist did not sign it. However, the signing radiologist also will be exposed to legal liability for obvious errors that occurred during the dictation or transcription process and should have been recognized in a thorough proofreading of the report (e.g., confusing statements, gross misspellings, or obvious omissions of words or sentences). Moreover, the signing radiologist might be liable for the incorrect interpretation of the dictating radiologist, on the grounds that the former had the opportunity to correct the error by looking at the radiographs but failed to do so.[19]

As Smith and Berlin recommend, "to obviate the need for signing a colleague's report, radiologists practicing in groups should consider using 'preliminary' or other temporary reports to give referring clinicians timely access to non-reviewed radiologic studies." Another approach is to utilize a system in which the clinician can hear the dictated report by dialing a telephone access number. Groups should consider providing laptop commuters to members who are on vacation so that they still can sign their reports even when away from work. Radiologists should sign a colleague's report only when a delay in final signing by the interpreting radiologist would be clearly unreasonable. In such circumstances, the signing radiologist should carefully proofread the report for obvious errors. There should be some indication in the report that it was signed by a radiologist other than the one interpreting it, possibly including the reason why the dictating radiologist was not available (such as due to illness). Although some have suggested signing the dictating radiologist's name, this could lead to disastrous accusations of cover-up or fraud if at trial it became apparent that the dictating radiologist actually was ill or on vacation at the time (without a laptop computer) and thus did not actually sign his or her name. If there is any suspicion of an underlying interpretive error, the signing radiologist should review the actual images, since he or she could well be exposed to legal liability.

Correction/Alteration of the Radiology Report

As with any medical record, alteration of a radiology report has serious consequences that can go far beyond the mere loss of a malpractice suit. "Once a radiology report is dictated, transcribed, signed by the radiologist, and sent out of the radiology department to physician's office or onto a patient's chart, that report should never be changed or withdrawn." If the radiologist wishes to make a change that reflects a new observation or interpretation, based on a review of the images or additional clinical information, he or she must dictate a revised report. This new report must be clearly identified as an "addendum" or "corrected" report. It should contain explicit language indicating that it supersedes the previous report and include the specific reason(s) why the initial report needed to be changed.[20]

Radiologists subjected to malpractice lawsuits may panic and consider making an addition or correction to an existing typed report to include material that might improve their legal positions. This is a foolhardy strategy that may have dire consequences. All physicians have a legal duty to maintain the integrity, accuracy, truth, and reliability of the patient's medical record.[21] Any deliberate falsification of the medical record by subsequent alteration, either by adding or deleting handwritten words or attempting to discard an incorrect initial typewritten report, could be construed as fraud and make the malpractice suit indefensible. Jurors who believe that a radiologist has tampered with records to cover up a mistake are highly likely to find the radiologist liable for malpractice, whether the specific medical facts support this finding.

Endnotes

1 Berlin L. Pitfalls of the vague radiology report. *AJR* 2000;174:1511–1518.
2 Berlin L. Malpractice issues in radiology: radiology reports. *AJR* 1997;169: 943–946.
3 American College of Radiology. ACR standard for communication: diagnostic radiology. In: *Standards 2000–2001*. Reston, VA: American College of Radiology,2001:3–5.
4 Spira R. Clinician, reveal thyself. *Appl Radiol* November 1996;5–13.
5 Rothman M. Malpractice issues in radiology: radiology reports (letter). *AJR* 1998;170:1108–1109.
6 Berlin L. Pitfalls of the vague radiology report. *AJR* 2000;174:1511–1518.
7 Naik SS, Hanbidge A, Wilson SR. Radiology reports: examining radiologist and clinical preferences regarding style and content. *AJR* 2001;176:591–598.
8 Lafortune M, Breton G, Baudouin JL. The radiological report; what is useful for the referring physician? *Can Assoc Radiol J* 1998;39:140–143.
9 Gunderman R, Ambrosius WT, Cohen M. Radiology reporting in an academic children's hospital: what referring physicians think. *Pediatr Radiol* 2000;30:307–314.
10 American College of Radiology. ACR standard for communication: diagnostic radiology. In: *Standards 2000–2001*. Reston, VA: American College of Radiology, 2001:3–5.
11 Berlin L. Pitfalls of the vague radiology report. *AJR* 2000;174:1511–1518.
12 Berlin L. Relying on the radiologist. *AJR* 2002;179:43–46.
13 *Medical-Legal Issues for Residents in Radiology*. Reston, VA: American College of Radiology, 1994:31–32.

14 Ibid.
15 Berlin L. Must new radiographs be compared with all previous radiographs, or only with the most recently obtained radiographs? *AJR* 2000;174:611–615.
16 Berlin L. Malpractice issues in radiology: comparing new radiographs with those obtained previously. *AJR* 1999;172:3–6.
17 *Blankshain v Radiology and Nuclear Consultants Ltd.*, 95L-4851 (Ill 1997).
18 Smith JJ, Berlin L. Signing a colleague's radiology report. *AJR* 2001;176:27–30.
19 *Jenoff v Gleason*, 521 A2d 1323 (NJ Super Ct App Div 1987).
20 Berlin L. Alteration of medical records. *AJR* 1997;168:1405–1408.
21 *In Re Jascalevich*, 442 A2d 635 (NJ App Ct, 1982).

17
Communication of the Radiologic Findings

Communication errors are the fourth most frequent primary allegation in malpractice lawsuits against radiologists.[1] According to the most recent American College of Radiology (ACR) standards,[2] "Communication is a critical component of the art and science of medicine and is especially important in diagnostic radiology. An official report (see prior section) shall be generated following any examination, procedure, or officially request consultation.... The final written report is considered to be the definitive means of communicating the results of an imaging examination or procedure to the referring physician.... Other methods for direct or personal communication of results are encouraged in certain situations. The timeliness of reporting any radiologic examination varies with the nature and urgency of the clinical problem." The following are some elements of communication that can lead to a malpractice lawsuit against a radiologist.

Failure to Issue a Report

Improper Patient Registration

To ensure that a report is dictated in every case, it is essential that technologists be instructed to follow rigid registration policies so that all radiologic examinations are accurately identified and presented to the radiologist for interpretation. Adherence to this guideline is especially important when breakdowns in this policy are likely to occur—with members of the medical staff or the radiologist's family, or studies performed on well-known entertainment or sports figures.[3] Except in dire emergencies, no patient should be examined without proper registration, even if the time delay causes some inconvenience. This rule is particularly important for examinations performed after normal working hours, when the radiologist on call has agreed to interpret every imaging study performed during that period even if he or she does not actually see them until the next day. In one case,[4] an emergency medicine physician asked to have a chest x-ray performed on himself, refused to register at the time due to time constraints, looked at the study himself and incorrectly read it as normal, and then placed the radiographs in a film jacket, which was filed away without the radiologist on call ever knowing of its existence. When the physician later developed a lung malignancy and there was evidence of the lesion on the initial film, a court deemed that there was a valid physician–patient relationship and thus the radiologist was subject to a malpractice lawsuit.

Similarly, it is essential to properly register and document any requests for interpretation of radiologic examinations from outside facilities. Such studies should be promptly presented to the radiologist for interpretation and the preparation of a formal written report.[5]

Improper Demographic Information

The ACR standards mandate that every radiograph be properly marked with the date and time of the examination. The written report should contain essential demographic data including, at a minimum, the names of the patient and referring physician, the type and date or the examination, and the dates of dictation and transcription.[6]

Delay in Issuing a Report[7]

Removal of Radiographs from the Radiology Department

Radiographs may be removed from the radiology department before the radiologist has an opportunity to interpret the study and dictate a written report. This is especially common in teaching hospitals, where house officers often sequester films to present to attending physicians at ward rounds or conferences and then fail to return them to the radiology department in a timely fashion. It is essential that a report indicating this removal of films be rendered promptly, using a phrase such as: "The radiographs have been removed from the department and thus are not available for interpretation at this time." If the images have been signed out before being interpreted and not returned, the name of the physician taking the films should be stated in the report. In addition to providing a reason why the radiologist has not met the ACR standard of rendering a written report in a "timely manner," this contemporaneously prepared explanation decreases the likelihood that in a subsequent lawsuit the plaintiff's attorney will charge (or a jury believe) that the radiologist deliberately destroyed a report to cover up an error (see page 129).

Incomplete Examination or Need to Obtain Old Films

The radiologist may require additional views, comparison with previous studies, or further clinical history before rendering a formal interpretation of an examination. However, one must avoid delaying an inordinate time in getting this information. Radiologists should establish a clear policy indicating a cutoff time at which a written report must be created, even if not all the relevant material is available. If additional pertinent information becomes available at a subsequent time, the radiologist can always issue an addendum to the original report, specifically indicating the reason for any differences from the initial interpretation. An open-ended wait for additional views, comparison studies, or clinical information runs the risk that the original films or requisition will be lost and increases the danger that no interpretation (even an admittedly incomplete one) will be rendered.

Direct Communication

To the Referring Physician

Failure to communicate urgent or significant unexpected findings directly to the referring physician is a major issue in almost 60% of malpractice lawsuits involving radiologists, even though in three quarters of them the medical record shows that a radiology report was issued in a timely manner.[8] In a more recent study, poor communication between providers of care resulted in the second highest average and third highest total amount of indemnification paid to plaintiffs.[9]

Traditionally, radiologists have seen themselves as "doctors' doctors"—consultants who performed radiologic examinations only on the request of a referring physician and then rendered a radiographic interpretation for, and transmitted to, the same physician.[10] Most radiologists believed that their duty to communicate interpretations was fulfilled by the sending of the official written report from the radiology department to the referring physician, with little concern about the possibility that the report might not be received or noticed by that physician in a timely fashion.[11]

In response to several court cases holding radiologists liable for failing to communicate radiographic results directly to a referring physician, the ACR (1991) issued its first Standard for Communication: Diagnostic Radiology. This noted the existence of certain circumstances that "may require direct communication of unusual, unexpected, or urgent findings to the referring physician in advance of a formal written report," concluding that "the timeliness of direct communication should be based upon the immediacy of the clinical situation." It is now well established that radiologists have a legal duty to directly communicate, either in person or by telephone, unexpected significant findings to the referring physician.[12] This includes the probable detection of "conditions carrying the risk of acute morbidity and/or mortality which may require immediate case management decisions" or "disease with non-acute morbidity or mortality sufficiently serious that it may require prompt notification of the patient, clinical evaluation, or initiation of treatment." Specific examples of situations in which direct communication may be indicated include radiologic diagnoses that necessitate immediate treatment decisions (e.g., pneumothorax, misplaced endotracheal or nasogastric tube); potentially life-threatening diagnoses (e.g., cancer of the breast, lung, or colon); conflict between emergency/preliminary and final reports; and potentially significant incidental findings made during other studies (e.g., lung mass on a preoperative chest radiograph).[13] The 2001 revision of the ACR standards[14] notes that "direct communication is accomplished in person or by telephone to the referring physician or an appropriate representative."

At times, foreseeable delays in the transmission of routine reports may require direct telephone communication to referring physicians of significant but not urgent findings that otherwise could travel through regular channels. Examples include long holiday weekends, on which no mail is delivered, and technical breakdowns in dictation or transcription equipment. Furthermore, direct communication is especially important when abnormalities are detected on "routine" examinations such as preoperative chest radiographs. Referring physicians are less likely to expect positive findings on such routine studies and often do not read the written reports, which also have an increased risk of getting lost in the system.[15]

Complying fully with this requirement can play havoc with the operations of a busy radiology department. The referring physician may not be clearly identified. Some patients are being evaluated by several consultants, so that the one who actually ordered the radiographic examination may not be the one to whom the report should best be communicated. Rightly or wrongly, surgeons may assume no responsibility for medical problems identified on preoperative imaging examinations, thus forcing the radiologist who detects an abnormality to track down the patient's internist or primary care physician.[16] Radiographs may be ordered by physicians who are not in the hospital network or even in the area, and accurate telephone numbers are often not available. In an increasingly hectic work environment, "it is not uncommon to spend

20–30 minutes trying to reach a 'body' only to find that the one who answers is unaware of anything about the patient, even if the patient is truly theirs." Moreover, radiologists frequently report cases long after the physician has left his or her office.[17] In an academic setting, a resident who ordered an examination may have rotated off the service, and the new resident may have no knowledge of the patient. The radiologist who decides that a finding must be reported via telephone must continue efforts to reach the referring physician or an acceptable alternate (such as a doctor who is covering for the primary physician) to complete the communication. Terminating attempts at communication because the referring physician is not easily available may place the radiologist in greater medical and legal jeopardy than not having attempted to telephone in the first place.[18]

One solution is to have a single person, such as a senior secretary, in each major department (e.g., medicine, surgery) whom the radiologist calls to report an urgent or unexpected significant finding. If the precise identity of the referring physician is unclear, this individual becomes responsible for obtaining the patient's chart and tracking down the appropriate physician to receive the verbal radiology report. If the secretary is not in the office, the radiologist can leave the pertinent information on an answering machine, under a prearranged agreement that the secretary will check for messages on a regular and frequent basis. In this way, the radiologist is obligated to make only a single telephone call, and disruptions in departmental flow are minimized as much as possible.

Whenever possible, it is essential that radiologists document in the formal written report that they have provided a direct verbal communication of the radiographic findings to the referring physician. Ideally, this documentation should include the name of the specific person contacted and the time when the communication was made. "If the verbal communication is completed after the radiology report has been dictated and signed, then the radiologist should keep a log in the department and document all pertinent discussions as they occur. An acceptable alternative would be to issue an addendum report that documents the [direct verbal] communication."[19]

To the Patient

In the past few years, there has been a definite trend toward expanding the duty of radiologists to communicate findings directly to patients. According to Berlin,[20] this phenomenon was initially generated by the courts "but is currently fueled by three sources—the federal government; the consumerism movement; and … 'entrepreneurial' radiology."

Courts have ruled that a radiologist must "take reasonable steps to make information available timely to the examinee of any findings that pose an imminent danger to the examinee's physical or mental well-being," concluding that "a physician's professional and ethical obligations imposed by the license to practice would demand no less."[21] The Mammography Quality Standards Act (1999) mandates that patients be sent a summary of the report written in lay terms within 30 days of a mammographic examination. In that same year, the ACR standards introduced the concept of direct communication to the patient, indicating that if the referring physician cannot be reached to report an urgent finding, "the interpreting physician should directly communicate the need for emergent care to the patient or responsible guardian, if possible," thus informing the patient to come to a hospital emergency room for immediate care.

The growing consumer movement and the desire of many patients to have more direct control over health care decisions have increased demand for direct communication of the results of radiographic studies. This has been abetted by the flourishing of imaging centers that provide screening examinations and directly inform patients of the results. As one advertisement in a popular magazine advised readers, "If you have a test, be sure to call and get the results. No news is not necessarily good news."[22]

Some radiologists[23] have gone so far as to recommend expanding the duty of members of their specialty to include discussing imaging findings with patients, presenting them with "clinical recommendation as to the course of action," suggesting "alternative behavior or life styles," and making an "appropriate referral when necessary." In this way, radiologists could "take a more dominant role in the health of our patients," thus becoming "not only a physicians' physician but also a patient's physician."

Placing the radiologist squarely in the clinical arena raises a host of potential medical-legal and political issues. Radiologists are trained to render interpretations of imaging studies, and most would probably feel uncomfortable if not inadequate in offering medical advice and participating in direct clinical management of patients. They would probably be held to the same standard of care as those who regularly perform direct patient care—internists and family practice physicians—who have years of intensive residency training in this area. Direct reporting of results to patients would require a large time commitment on the part of radiologists, who would need to explain the results and to answer questions from patients and patients' families, people with whom radiologists would otherwise have no personal contact. In all probability, courts would still require direct communication of urgent and significant unexpected findings to referring physicians, thus duplicating the demands on already overstressed and overworked radiologists. Finally, many referring physicians who have historically believed that only they should transmit radiology results to their patients might resent radiologists' attempting to communicate results directly to their patients. Although this is currently the case under the Mammography Quality Standards Act, referring physicians had no choice but to accept the mandatory government-imposed rules; most would probably not so easily accept the concept of direct communication of results to patients having other imaging studies if they were adopted unilaterally by radiologists.[24]

The costs and difficulties of implementing a system of directly communicating results of radiologic examinations to patients and the potential danger of souring relations with referring physicians might have one underlying benefit—the reduction, if not the elimination, of malpractice lawsuits alleging failure to communicate urgent or significant radiographic abnormalities. This has occurred with respect to mammographic examinations following the mandatory reporting requirements imposed by the Mammography Quality Standards Act. However, radiologists who also choose to advise patients on treatment options or other aspects of clinical management would be raising the specter of a new type of malpractice lawsuit alleging breaches of the standard of care in an area for which most have not been adequately prepared in residency training programs.[25]

Endnotes

1 Physician Insurers Association of America and American College of Radiology. *Practice Standards Claims Survey*. Rockville, MD: Physician Insurers Association of America, 1997.

2 American College of Radiology. ACR standard for communication: diagnostic radiology. In: *Standards 2000--2001*. Reston, VA: American College of Radiology, 2001:3—5.

3 Berlin L. The importance of patient registration and processing. *AJR* 1997; 169:1483–1486.

4 *Grossman v Los Alamitas Medical Center*, 635386 (Orange County, Cal 1993).

5 Berlin L. The importance of patient registration and processing. *AJR* 1997; 169:1483–1486.

6 Ibid.

7 Ibid.

8 Physician Insurers Association of America and American College of Radiology. *Practice Standards Claims Survey*. Rockville, MD: Physician Insurers Association of America, 1997.

9 Physician Insurers Association of America (unpublished data).cited in Berlin *AJR* 2002;178:809–815.

10 Berlin L. The radiologist: doctor's doctor or patient's doctor? (Editorial) *AJR* 1977;128:702.

11 Robertson CL, Kopans DB. Communications problems after mammographic screening. *Radiology* 1989;172:443–444.

12 Cascade PN, Berlin L. American College of Radiology standard for communication. *AJR* 1999;173:1439–1442

13 *Medical-Legal Issues for Residents in Radiology*. Reston, VA: American College of Radiology, 1994:22.

14 American College of Radiology: ACR standard for communication: diagnostic radiology. In: *Standards 2000–2001*. Reston, VA: American College of Radiology, 2001:3–5.

15 Berlin L. Communication of the significant but not urgent finding. *AJR* 1997;168:329–331.

16 Berlin L. Communicating findings of radiologic examinations: Whither goest the radiologist's duty? *AJR* 2002;178:809–815.

17 Dalinka MK. Communication, the deep pocket, and ACR standards (letter). *AJR* 2001;177:248.

18 Berlin L. Communicating findings of radiologic examinations: Whither goest the radiologist's duty? *AJR* 2002;178:809–815.

19 Berlin L. Communication of the urgent finding. *AJR* 1996;166:513–516.

20 Berlin L. Communicating findings of radiologic examinations: Whither goest the radiologist's duty? *AJR* 2002;178:809–815.

21 *Ranier v Frieman*, 682 A2d 1220 (NJ App 1996).

22 How to prevent medical errors: major causes of death in the United States. People, July 2, 2001:16–17.

23 Bluth EI. A new paradigm for radiology. *Decisions in Imaging Economics* 2001;16(6):9.

24 Berlin L. Communicating findings of radiologic examinations: Whither goest the radiologist's duty? *AJR* 2002;178:809–815.

25 Ibid.

18
Release and Storage of Radiologic Images

Ownership of Images

Courts have generally regarded radiologic images, as well as other medical records, as the property of the health care facility in which they were produced. Nevertheless, state laws guarantee access to the radiologic images by the patient or other physicians engaged in the patient's care, though they do not have a right to possess the originals. Patients often fail to appreciate the distinction between ownership of a tangible film and the information it contains—that in essence they are paying for the professional service of the radiologist rather than the physical recording device upon which it is based.[1] Consequently, the patient cannot use the radiologist's retention of the images as a defense to a suit to collect professional fees.[2]

Patient Access to Images

The health care institution must provide the patient with access to his or her radiologic images and other medical records. Furthermore, upon valid authorization by the patient, a radiology facility must release images and reports to other physicians involved in the clinical care of the patient. Most radiology departments subscribe to a policy of retaining the original images, releasing only copies to the patient or referring physicians. State laws permit patients to be charged the cost of duplicating radiologic images or reports; however, in the face of a strong protest by the patient, it is advisable to reduce or even waive the fee to maintain good will.[3]

Refusal of a patient's request for inspection or valid release of films (or any other medical record) can have serious consequences. Courts or administrative agencies can impose stiff fines, state medical boards can take disciplinary action for unprofessional conduct, and the patient may even institute a lawsuit based on a claim of fraudulent conceal-ment. An exception is a case in which physicians can produce evidence supporting their belief that release of such records can harm the pa-tient.[4]

Once radiologists are informed, or reasonably believe, that specific radiographic studies may be the subject of a lawsuit, they must take extra precautions to ensure that the original images are preserved. Under these circumstances, original images should not be released with-out a court order.[5]

Some radiology departments feel that the additional expense of copy-ing all radiologic images before release is not warranted, and therefore they freely lend original radiographs when requested. When using this approach, Berlin[6] recommends that the patient sign a document that acknowledges the radiologic images as the property of the facility, and that contains the patient's name and other pertinent personal data, the specific radiologic images released and their destination, the date of the release of the images, and the requested date for their return. He of-fers the following sample statement: "I understand that these radiologic images are the legal property of X Hospital, and that they are being released to me on loan for the express purpose of having another phy-sician review them for medical purposes. Since these radiologic images are a part of the permanent records of X Hospital, I will return them within 90 days."

Radiologists should realize that the loss of original films, especially if copies are not made, may result in physicians or the facility, or both, falling out of compliance with state and federal retention laws. More-over, "comparison with previous studies becomes impossible; defense of medical malpractice lawsuits becomes difficult; reimbursement may be denied for rendered services; and litigation based on deliberate or negligent destruction (called 'spoliation') of evidence may arise" (see below). Therefore, most authorities recommend that facilities should never release original films except in response to a valid written re-quest by the patient or to a court order.[7]

Occasionally, radiologic images may have to be released before they have been interpreted officially. This generally occurs in a hospital when a patient admitted to the emergency department after normal working hours must be transferred to another facility after initial radiologic im-ages have been obtained. The next morning, a radiologist should dictate a formal report indicating that images obtained at the hospital were released without being interpreted. This prevents the scenario in which, in a malpractice lawsuit claiming negligence in diagnosis, the radiologic images are located but no interpretation can be found. When the radi-ologist states that he or she never actually saw the images and thus could not have rendered an interpretation, the plaintiff could charge that an interpretation was made but subsequently was found to be incorrect and then was deliberately lost. The potential legal pitfall can be avoided by having in the record a contemporaneous statement that the radiologic images were removed from the department before interpretation.[8]

Confidentiality

State and federal law, as well as the concept of physician–patient privilege, mandate that patient medical records be kept confidential. Although there are specific exceptions that permit or even require the release of information in cases of cancer, infectious disease, suspected child abuse, alcohol or drug abuse, and medical research, the "unauthorized breach of confidentiality exposes physicians and facilities to patient-initiated lawsuits for invasion of privacy, defamation, and negligent or intentional infliction of emotional distress." In addition, failure to maintain confidentiality may result in administrative fines and disciplinary actions imposed by state medical boards.

Consequently, before the release of any medical records, the patient should be required to sign a general or blanket waiver in which he or she agrees to limit potential liability related to any unintended or unauthorized use of such records. As noted above, the waiver also should specify where the records are going as well as their prospective use.[9]

Retention of Images

Laws governing the retention of radiographic images vary from state to state. Medicare and most states require that all medical records (including radiologic images) be kept for at least five years. However, it is strongly recommended to follow the American College of Radiology (ACR) guidelines that radiologic images be retained for at least an additional time period equal to the maximum period that the state statute of limitations permits the filing of a medical malpractice lawsuit.[10] This statute of limitations (see page 15), which runs from the time when a person knows or should know of the existence of an injury, is most commonly two years. Therefore, most radiologic facilities tend to retain images on adults for seven years (five plus two).

Some federal statutes require longer retention of images for specific types of examinations. "The Mammography Quality Standards Act [MQSA][11] requires the facility to retain mammograms and associated patient records for not less than 5 years, and not less than 10 years if no more mammograms of the patient have been obtained at the facility. The MQSA permits longer retention time if so specified by state statute, and its provisions are obviated when a patient requests the permanent transfer of records to another medical institution or physician, or to the patient herself." The Occupational Safety and Health Administration (OSHA) requires that the records of a patient exposed to toxic substances or harmful agents be retained for 30 years.[12] In addition, both federal and state statutes of limitation are extended if the injured party is a minor, disabled, imprisoned, or the victim of fraudulent concealment. [13]

In addition to patient care concerns, the retention of radiologic images is vital to ensure that they are available if a radiologist is sued for a missed diagnosis. An inability to find the images in the face of legal action is a potentially devastating situation that gives rise to the *spoliation* rule. This states that when evidence is lost, destroyed, or suppressed, a jury is entitled to presume that the missing evidence would be unfavorable to the party responsible for its unavailability (even if contrary evidence is produced that the images or other medical records would not have aided the plaintiff's case). Since diagnostic images are deemed to be under the control of the radiologist and the health care institution, an inability to produce pertinent images allows the jury to infer that the radiologist deliberately destroyed them because he or she had something to hide—a scenario that typically results in a verdict in favor of the plaintiff. Some jurisdictions have even recognized an independent tort of spoliation of evidence.[14] At times, the spoliation rule can aid the radiologist-defendant in a malpractice suit. If the patient has signed out the original radiologic images and subsequently lost them, the presumption is that they would have been favorable to the defense, and the jury may decide for the defense despite otherwise damaging facts in the case.

Storage and Destruction of Images[15]

Radiology facilities generally store films in a local file room or in an off-site location. Most state and federal laws permit storage on microfilm, as long as a readable copy of the microfilmed record can be made available when necessary. [Storage of digital images in a filmless PACS system and via teleradiology is discussed on page 215.]

Medical records, including films, must be destroyed in accordance with an established plan. Burning or shredding of records, including radiology reports, may be required by state law, which also may mandate making an abstract of the pertinent data to be kept in the permanent record. The American Medical Association recommends, and many states require, that patients be notified before destruction of their records and offered the option of having the record retrieved and placed under their own control. Although it is common practice to resell old film to vendors for the reclaiming of silver, radiologists should be certain that such procedures are coordinated with applicable state statutes.

Endnotes

1 Brenner RJ, Westenberg L. Film management and custody: current and future medicolegal issues. *AJR* 1996;167:1371–1375.
2 Miller RD, Hutton RC. *Problems in Health Care Law, 8th ed.* Gaithersburg (MD), Aspen, 2000, pg. 534–535.
3 Berlin L. Storage and release of radiographs. *AJR* 1997;168:895–897.
4 Brenner RJ, Westenberg L. Film management and custody: current and future medicolegal issues. *AJR* 1996;167:1371–1375.
5 Berlin L. Storage and release of radiographs. *AJR* 1997;168:895–897.
6 Ibid.
7 Brenner RJ, Westenberg L. Film management and custody: current and future medicolegal issues. *AJR* 1996;167:1371–1375.
8 Berlin L. Storage and release of radiographs. *AJR* 1997;168:895–897.
9 Brenner RJ, Westenberg L. Film management and custody: current and future medicolegal issues. *AJR* 1996;167:1371–1375.
10 American College of Radiology. *ACR Digest of Council Actions.* Reston, VA: *ACR*, 1994:233–235.
11 42 USC 263B; 21 CFR #900.12(c)(4)(i,ii).
12 24 CFR #1910.20.
13 Brenner RJ, Westenberg L. Film management and custody: current and future medicolegal issues. *AJR* 1996;167:1371–1375.
14 Miller RD, Hutton RC. *Problems in Health Care Law, 8th ed.* Gaithersburg (MD), Aspen, 2000, pg. 543.
15 Brenner RJ, Westenberg L. Film management and custody: current and future medicolegal issues. *AJR* 1996;167:1371–1375.

19
Medical Records

Importance of Proper Medical Records[1]

As interventional procedures expand the role of the radiologist in the diagnosis and treatment of an increasing number of medical conditions, entries written into the hospital chart become more significant. Complete and accurate medical records are invaluable in malpractice lawsuits and may prove to be the radiologist's best defense. A good record suggests that the radiologist exercised due care in diagnosis and treatment of the patient, whereas a poor record may force settlement of a malpractice claim even when the case would otherwise be defensible.

Entries in the medical record are often the major mechanism for various members of the health care team to communicate with each other or with other medical facilities. Incomplete medical records can lead to irreparable injuries to patients and subsequent litigation. The radiologist should exercise great care in choosing descriptive terms, entering numbers and decimal points properly, and recording events. It is essential to use consistent terminology so that everyone has an accurate conception of what has occurred. Because other physicians may depend on what is written in the medical record, all entries must be legible, clear, and concise. Illegible records that cannot be properly deciphered may have grave consequences. All events occurring during the course of treatment should be entered promptly into the medical record with the time, the date, and a signature. Noting relevant telephone conversations in the medical record can be vitally important if there is later a dispute as to whether a conversation took place and what was said. At trial, a plaintiff's attorney will have great difficulty convincing a jury that his or her client's recollection of a conversation was more accurate than the physician's contemporaneous written notation of the conversation in the patient's medical record.

Correction/Alteration of the Medical Record

Alteration of a medical record has serious consequences that can go far beyond the mere loss of a malpractice suit. Once the entry is complete, changes or alterations should ordinarily not be made.[2]

If the radiologist later realizes that the initial entry contained a minor error, it is permissible to make a correction by placing a single line through the incorrect information (leaving the words legible), initialing or signing the correction, and entering the time and date of the correction. An incorrect entry should never be obliterated or erased, nor should a page of the record that contains erroneous and corrected entries ever be destroyed, for these actions may lead jurors to suspect the original entry and seriously decrease the credibility of the radiologist.[3] Under no circumstances should a radiologist add words or phrases to an existing entry at a later date. If it becomes apparent that the initial entry contained a more substantial error of fact or opinion, the radiologist should indicate this in an entirely new entry, documented with the later time or date.

Adverse Consequences of Improper Alteration of a Medical Record

Radiologists subjected to malpractice lawsuits may panic and consider making an addition or correction to an existing handwritten medical record (or typed report) to include material that might improve their legal positions. This is a bad strategy that may lead to a legal nightmare. All physicians have a legal duty to maintain "the integrity, accuracy, truth, and reliability of the patient's medical record."[4] Any deliberate falsification of the medical record by subsequent alteration—either by adding or deleting handwritten words or attempting to discard an incorrect initial typewritten report—could be construed as fraud and make the malpractice lawsuit indefensible. Changes or inconsistencies in the record, as well as destroyed or mutilated records, only suggest to a jury that the record has been altered because the physician has something to hide. Jurors who believe that a radiologist has tampered with records to cover up a mistake are highly likely to find the radiologist liable for malpractice, whether the specific medical facts support this finding, and to increase the size of a damage award.

Document examination is now a sophisticated science. By analyzing the pen and ink used, as well as the handwriting, experts may be able to determine precisely the time that entries were made in medical records and who made them. As a general rule, any attempt to "enhance" the medical record will prove to be more detrimental than helpful in defending a radiologist in a malpractice lawsuit. "Records with obvious alterations, particularly any record that can be shown to be 'fudged,'" are absolutely deadly in court.[5]

Improper alteration of a medical record can have effects far beyond the mere loss of a malpractice lawsuit. Because courts have regarded such actions as "gross malpractice endangering the health or life of the patient,"[6] improper alterations in medical records can result not only in compensatory damage but also in large punitive awards, which are not covered by professional liability insurance and must be paid personally by the physician.[7] In some states, a physician who improperly alters a medical record is subject to license revocation or other discipline for unprofessional conduct.[8] An insurance company may refuse to renew professional liability coverage. In some states, it is a crime to deliberately falsify a medical record. "Attempting to influence the outcome of a case, civil or criminal, by such methods as altering records under subpoena, or which are likely to be subject to subpoena, is a criminal offense." Altering or falsifying a medical record to obtain reimbursement wrongfully, such as by changing the date that a procedure was performed, is a crime.[9]

Inappropriate Entries[10]

Although not exposing one to civil or criminal penalties, certain statements are clearly inappropriate in a medical record (or formal radiology report). Radiologists must always remember that the purpose of medical records is to provide a written record of diagnoses and treatments and the facts and reasoning behind them, not as a soapbox for sarcastic comments. Nonprofessional opinions placed in the record endanger its credibility. Careless talk, open disputes, and second-guessing among colleagues regarding patient care can often lead to unwarranted malpractice actions. Thus, medical records should never be used to convey to colleagues "editorial comments" of potential legal significance relating to fellow physicians ("Dr. X has made another error") or to the patient ("She just complains all the time; not sick but crazy").

The medical record and radiology report should only contain necessary objective facts; criticisms of other physicians, witticisms, and derogatory or indiscreet remarks must be avoided. But if such comments are recorded in a moment of weakness, one should never attempt to tamper with or alter them. The lesser of two evils is to simply leave them alone, "except for an explanation as to the genesis of the error and an appropriate retraction."

Endnotes

1 *Medical-Legal Issues for Residents in Radiology.* Reston, VA: American College of Radiology, 1994:35–38.
2 Berlin L. Alteration of medical records. *AJR* 1997;168:1405–1408.
3 Miller RD, Hutton RC. *Problems in Health Care Law, 8th ed.* Gaithersburg (MD), Aspen, 2000, pg. 540.
4 In Re Jascalevich, 442 A2d 635 (NJ App Ct, 1982).
5 Buckner F. Medical records and disclosure about patients. In: Sanbar SS, Gibofsky A, Firestone MH, et al (eds). *Legal Medicine, 5th ed.* St. Louis, Mosby, 2001, pg 270.
6 Ibid.
7 Rice B. "Doctoring" a chart cost this M.D. $1 million. *Med Econ* 1996;78–92.
8 Miller RD, Hutton RC. *Problems in Health Care Law, 8th ed.* Gaithersburg (MD), Aspen, 2000, pg. 541.
9 Buckner F. Medical records and disclosure about patients. In: Sanbar SS, Gibofsky A, Firestone MH, et al (eds). *Legal Medicine, 5th ed.* St. Louis, Mosby, 2001, pg 270.
10 Ibid.

20
Confidentiality

Medical information that patients give to their doctors and hospital staff contains a wealth of personal health care history as well as demographic, sexual, behavioral, dietary, and recreational data. Because of the vast amount of highly sensitive information that their medical record contains, patients reasonably expect that it will be kept strictly private.[1] The sacrosanct nature of the confidentiality of the physician-patient relationship dates back to antiquity. The Hippocratic Oath (4th century B.C.E.) unequivocally requires the physician to swear that "all that may come to my knowledge in the exercise of my profession or outside of my profession or in daily commerce with men, which ought not to be spread abroad ... I will never reveal. If I keep this oath faithfully, may I enjoy my life and practice my art, respected by all men and in all times; but if I swerve from it or violate it, may the reverse be my lot." This strict requirement for keeping patient information in confidence remains a basic ethical principle.[2] As the Code of Medical Ethics of the American Medical Association states: "In most states, either by statute or case law, disclosure of medical information is prohibited without the consent of the patient.... Patients must be able to secure medical services without fear of betrayal and unwarranted embarrassing and detrimental disclosure of private information." Nevertheless, the code adds that some "overriding social consideration" will make revelations "ethically and legally justified."[3] Confidential medical information can be disclosed without patient consent for public health and health oversight activities, judicial and administrative proceedings, coroners and medical examiners, law enforcement and research purposes, government health data systems, and in emergency situations.[4]

The huge amounts of health information electronically shuttled around the world in computer banks, for such purposes as billing, quality management, statistical analysis, and research, have made it inevitable that there be notorious incidents in which patient confidentiality has been violated or ignored. A large Royal Commission of Inquiry in Ontario, Canada, as well as other studies worldwide, "revealed widespread abuses of patient confidentiality by attorneys, insurance companies, and government agencies." Given the devastating effects that inappropriate disclosures may have on patients, as well as the ever-increasing spread of this information by electronic means, there has been a resurgence of interest in a comprehensive federal law governing the confidentiality of medical records.[5]

In 1996, Congress passed the Kennedy-Kassebaum bill,[6] also known as the Health Insurance Portability and Accountability Act (HIPAA), which called for the enactment of a privacy statute within three years. Despite recommendations for the framework of such legislation provided by the secretary of health and human services, Congress failed to enact a comprehensive health care privacy law. Instead, it instructed the secretary to develop a set of proposed regulations, which were published in November 1999.[7] These extremely complex and controversial regulations have engendered fierce debate but are now law. These rules apply only to health plans, health care clearinghouses (e.g., billing and collection agencies, accountants), and health care providers who transmit health information *electronically*. Thus paper and film records are not covered, and nonprovider, nonplan, and nonclearinghouse holders of health care information are not included.[8] Moreover, the Compliance and Enforcement section does not allow for a private action against violators, nor does it prescribe specific penalties that the secretary may impose.[9]

The following are among the major provisions of the proposed rules[10]:

a. requires a written authorization from the patient to release information to a health care entity, a non-health-care-related division of the same entity, or the patient's employer[11]
b. requires notice to patients of the entity's information practices[12]
c. allows patients to access and copy their medical records[13]
d. provides patients with an accounting of disclosures except those for treatment, payment, and health care operations, and those to health oversight or law enforcement agencies[14]
e. allows patients to make amendments and corrections to medical records[15]
f. requires the covered entities to designate an individual responsible for privacy issues, have a contact person or office, train personnel in health information policies, and have in place administrative, technical, and physical safeguards for health care information[16]
g. requires documentation of all policies and procedures and retention of that documentation for at least 6 years[17]
h. requires all covered entities to be in compliance within 2 years of the effective date of the regulations[18]

HIPAA requires that health care providers ensure the confidentiality, integrity, and availability of patient health information (PHI). *Integrity* refers to making certain that information is not damaged, corrupted, or destroyed; a*vailability* means that the information must be made continuously available to those authorized to have it whenever it is needed. Steps to protect the privacy and electronic security of health information include never sharing passwords, logging off computer stations when finished, shredding written records that are no longer needed (not leaving it in a trash bin), enforcing the use of security and visitor badges, always encrypting e-mail messages and adding a confidentiality statement noting that the material is only for the use of designated recipients, and never faxing information to an unsecured fax machine (located in a nonrestricted environment).[19]

HIV-Positive Patients

The early stages of the AIDS epidemic in the late 1980s and early 1990s led to the enactment of state laws concerning the confidentiality of HIV-related information.[20] Most of these cases involved homosexual men and IV drug users, groups who long have been subjected to discrimination. In view of the widespread public fear of what was perceived to be an untreatable, universally fatal illness, advocates for HIV-positive patients argued that easy access to HIV-status information would discourage those at risk from being tested.[21] As one court noted, "even though most Americans understand the modes through which HIV is spread, a significant minority still would exclude those who are HIV-positive from schools, public accommodations and the work place. Unauthorized disclosure of a person's serologic status can lead to social opprobrium among family and friends, as well as loss of employment, housing and insurance."[22]

Although laws to protect the confidentiality of HIV-related information vary widely from state to state,[23] they typically require informed consent for HIV testing and strict confidentiality of test results. Nevertheless, access to results is permitted in limited circumstances, which usually involve threats to public health.[24,25]

Radiologists must be scrupulously careful to keep information concerning the HIV status of their patients strictly confidential, permitting access only to those health care professionals directly involved in these patients' care. They also must warn technologists and support staff of the serious consequences that may result from the unauthorized disclosure of such information. Similarly, health care facilities must establish meaningful policies or procedures that provide all reasonable measures necessary to limit access to medical charts so as to ensure patient confidentiality.[26]

In certain circumstances, a demonstrated threat to public health requiring disclosure of HIV status may override a patient's personal right to privacy. In one case, an obstetrics-gynecology resident accidentally cut during a surgical procedure underwent a blood test that revealed he was HIV-positive. Believing that the resident might have exposed patients and members of the staff to the virus, the medical center convinced the court to allow disclosure. In response to the resident's appeal, a higher court confirmed the ruling, observing that "individual privacy interests in medical information and records are not absolute. At times, the societal interest in disclosure outweighs the individual's interest in privacy. To avoid a constitutional violation, the state must show a compelling interest for breaching the privacy right. Here, the risk of transmission of a fatal disease and the prevention of the spread of AIDS are both appropriate state interests."[27] By extension, the results in this case would seem applicable to radiologists and residents involved in interventional studies.

Endnotes

1 Buckner F. Medical records and disclosure about patients. In: Sanbar SS, Gibofsky A, Firestone MH, et al (eds). *Legal Medicine, 5th ed*. St. Louis, Mosby, 2001, pg 273.

2 Smith JJ, Berlin L. The HIV-positive patient and confidentiality. *AJR* 2001;176:599–602.

3 AMA Council on Ethical and Judicial Affairs. *Code of Medical Ethics: Current Opinions and Annotations*, #5.05 (1997).

4 Standards for Privacy of Individually Identifiable Health Information: Proposed Rule, 64 Federal Register 59917 at 59919, Section 164.510 (November 3, 1999).

5 Carlisle JR. Ethics and bioethics. In: Sanbar SS, Gibofsky A, Firestone MH, et al (eds). *Legal Medicine, 5th ed*. St. Louis, Mosby, 2001, pgs 293–294.

6 Health Insurance Portability and Accountability Act of 1996, 42 U.S.C. #1320.

7 Standards for Privacy of Individually Identifiable Health Information: Proposed Rule, 64 Federal Register 59917 at 59919 (November 3, 1999).

8 Ibid., Section 160.102.

9 Ibid., Section 164.522.

10 Buckner F. Medical records and disclosure about patients. In: Sanbar SS, Gibofsky A, Firestone MH, et al (eds). *Legal Medicine, 5th ed*. St. Louis, Mosby, 2001, pgs , 275–276.

11 Standards for Privacy of Individually Identifiable Health Information: Proposed Rule, 64 Federal Register 59917 at 59919 (November 3, 1999), Section 164.508.

12 Ibid., Section 164.510.

13 Ibid., Section 164.514.

14 Ibid., Section 164.515.

15 Ibid., Section 164.516.

16 Ibid., Section 164.518.

17 Ibid., Section 164.520.

18 Ibid., Section 164.524.

19 *UCSF HIPAA Handbook*. San Francisco: University of California at San Francisco, January 2003.

20 Doughty R. *The confidentiality of HIV-related information: responding to the resurgence of aggressive public health interventions in the AIDS epidemic*. 82 Calif L Rev 111:1994.

21 Smith JJ, Berlin L. The HIV-positive patient and confidentiality. *AJR* 2001; 176:599–602.

22 *Behringer v Medical Center at Princeton*, 592 A2d 1251 (NJ Sup Ct 1991).

23 Taylor J. *Sex, lies, and lawsuits: a New Mexico physician's duty to warn third parties who unknowingly may be at risk of contracting HIV from a patient*. 26 NM L Rev 481:1996.

24 Doughty R. *The confidentiality of HIV-related information: responding to the resurgence of aggressive public health interventions in the AIDS epidemic*. 82 Calif L Rev 111:1994.

25 *In re: Application of the Milton S. Hershey Medical Center of the PA State University, Appeal of John Doe, MD*, 595 A2d 1290 (PA Super Ct 1991).

26 Smith JJ, Berlin L. The HIV-positive patient and confidentiality. *AJR* 2001;176:599–602.

27 *In re: Application of the Milton S. Hershey Medical Center of the PA State University, Appeal of John Doe, MD*, 595 A2d 1290 (PA Super Ct 1991).

Part IV
Radiology Practice and Specific Procedures

21
Consent

It is a well-established principle that, in the absence of a serious emergency, a physician must obtain consent before examining a patient or performing a diagnostic or therapeutic procedure. As clearly enunciated by Benjamin Cardozo in 1914,[1] an adult of sound mind has the right to decide what shall be done with his or her own body. Traditionally, failure to obtain consent from a patient before instituting medical care exposed a physician to a charge of *battery*, which is defined legally as the intentional harmful or offensive touching of another person without authorization. The mere touching without permission is sufficient to incur liability, even if the procedure is performed properly, beneficial, and without any negative effects. As an intentional tort, battery may not be covered under a professional liability policy. It also could expose a physician to punitive damages, additional awards intended not only to provide restitution to the injured party but also to punish the offending party and deter similar behavior in the future. Obtaining any consent to the procedure, even if not fully informed (see below), defeats the claim of battery.

Today, the absence of appropriate consent is actionable under the principle of *negligence*, in which the physician is held to the standard of "reasonableness" according to one of two standards (see below).

Types of Consent

Consent may be either express or implied. Express consent is given by direct words, either oral or written, in which the patient specifically grants the physician permission to undertake the diagnosis or treatment of a particular problem. Because oral consent is difficult to prove in court, virtually all physicians seek written consent.

Implied consent is inferred from the conduct of the patient. Examples include a patient voluntarily climbing onto a radiography table or drinking a barium solution. Courts have established two prerequisites for a finding of consent implied by voluntary submission. First, the patient must have some comprehension of the nature of the proposed procedure or treatment and be made aware of the common risks associated with it. Second, the patient must have an opportunity to withdraw from the procedure or treatment. Relying on a patient's implied consent poses a substantial legal risk and should be reserved only for simple procedures, such as ordinary radiographic examinations and most noninvasive studies. Although simply extending an arm to receive an intravenous injection of contrast material could be construed as implied consent, the radiologist should nevertheless clearly explain to the patient the benefits and risks of the procedure.

Consent is *presumed* to exist in medical emergencies, unless the provider has reason to believe that consent would be refused. When unexpected emergency conditions arise during an interventional procedure, especially if life threatening, implied consent may be found to extend to modifications of the procedure beyond the scope expressly authorized. If time permits, however, the radiologist should wait and obtain consent for the additional procedure. For example, if the patient has consented to a peripheral arteriogram that demonstrates a stenotic lesion amenable to balloon dilatation, the radiologist should not proceed to an angioplasty without securing additional consent. Other situations in which implied consent is presumed include the minor child who requires urgent care, comatose patients needing immediate treatment, the mentally incompetent, the unavailability of a legal guardian, and the intoxicated patient who temporarily lacks the capacity to reason (i.e., consent).[2]

Informed Consent

Modern law considers the decision whether to undergo a diagnostic or therapeutic procedure to be a joint decision between the physician and a patient who possesses enough information to enable an intelligent choice. Although often considered as a mere administrative burden, "physicians who actually engage in the intended communication with their patients find that it not only performs its intended function of respecting individual autonomy, but also improves compliance, outcomes, and satisfaction."[3]

Courts have developed two basic standards for determining whether disclosure of information is adequate to meet the requirements of informed consent. The traditional approach is the *reasonable physician* standard ("majority rule") of accepted medical practice. States following this principle require that the physician disclose the risks of a procedure to a degree commensurate with the prevailing practice of reasonable medical practitioners under the same or similar circumstances. Expert testimony is necessary to prove what the reasonable physician would be required to disclose to the patient.[4]

The newer approach, adopted by about half the states, is the *reasonable patient* standard ("minority rule").[5] This mandates that the physician disclose all "material" risks—information that the reasonable patient would want to know before deciding whether or not to undergo the proposed diagnostic or therapeutic procedure. The disclosure should be tailored to the ability of the patient to comprehend, since it is designed to affect the patient's decision-making process. Using this standard, there is no need for expert testimony concerning the scope of disclosure, though expert testimony is generally necessary to prove the existence of risks and alternatives.[6] In practice, there often is little substantial difference between these two standards. In states with the reasonable physician standard, the plaintiff can usually find an expert witness willing to testify that the defendant radiologist failed to obtain appropriate consent. Juries may bend over backward to accept such testimony despite contrary evidence given by an expert witness for the defense, viewing with suspicion and distaste what they deem the arrogant and paternalistic attitude of a radiologist who does not provide all the information that the patient needs to make a reasonable decision.[7]

Regardless of the standard used, patients should be made to understand that it is impossible to guarantee a perfect outcome and that every procedure has inherent risks. The chance of a poor outcome unrelated to the quality of care is possible in virtually every medical encounter. The radiologist obtaining informed consent should remember that prior to a procedure a patient is under a great deal of stress and may not fully grasp the situation. Therefore, it may be beneficial during the process of informed consent to summarize the information in writing and allow the patient and the family some time to review and digest all that has been explained. The radiologist can then return and answer any additional questions before having the patient sign a formal consent form.

Informed consent rarely becomes an issue as long as the procedure was successfully completed without any complications resulting in patient injury. Conversely, "obtaining legally adequate informed consent merely confirms that a patient voluntarily submitted to a test or procedure. The doctrine provides no protection against subsequent negligence in the performance of that test or procedure." Therefore, even the most thorough informed consent provides no shield against a malpractice lawsuit.[8]

What Radiographic Procedures Require Consent?

The American College of Radiology recommends that informed consent be obtained from patients who are to undergo radiologic procedures "with a significant incidence of serious complications," but does not specifically define this phrase. In the classic case of *Canterbury*,[9] the physician was held liable for failure to divulge a 1% risk of paralysis associated with a laminectomy. However, the court stressed the serious nature of the undisclosed risk rather than the mathematical possibility of its occurrence.[10] Virtually all in the radiology community agree that informed consent must be obtained for all interventional procedures. However, there is no clear policy for less invasive studies, such as those requiring the intravenous injection of iodinated contrast material. Nevertheless, in view of a case[11] holding that failure to inform a patient of the risks surrounding the administration of contrast material was virtually equivalent to a declaration that there were no risks, it is reasonable to inform patients undergoing contrast studies of the small, but real, risk of a potentially serious reaction. Pretest screening for risk factors may identify potential problems. "If a patient has identifiable risk factors for contrast reaction or has poor renal function, the increased risk of an adverse reaction or of contrast agent-induced renal failure should be communicated to the patient."[12]

Elements of Disclosure

Under either the reasonable physician or reasonable patient standard, the radiologist should explain to the patient (a) the diagnosis and nature of the condition or illness calling for medical intervention; (b) the nature and purpose of the proposed procedure (benefits); (c) its known material risks and potential complications; (d) the relative probability of success for the treatment of procedure stated in understandable terms; (e) all available reasonable and acceptable alternatives to the procedure (including their material risks and potential complications); and (f) the probable outcome if no procedure or treatment is performed.[13]

The courts have indicated that not all risks are material, but they have not provided any specific indication of how to determine which ones must be disclosed to the patient. In general, the radiologist should disclose those risks that have the most severe consequences and those that have a substantial probability of occurring. Radiologists do not need to disclose precise percentages of risks or the odds of success of a given procedure[14]; however, if they do volunteer such statistics and they are substantially wrong, there could be liability for misstatements.[15]

All information must be in language that the patient can understand; an explanation in technical terms incomprehensible to the patient does not constitute informed consent.[16]

For interventional therapeutic procedures, disclosure should include a realistic discussion of the likelihood of success from the proposed treatment, as well as the alternatives of no treatment or "conservative" treatment. It is important to make certain that the patient does not construe an explanation of the hoped-for benefits of the procedure as a promise or guarantee. The radiologist should be sensitive to the occupation and hobbies of the patient, since specific complications could have a substantially more devastating effect depending on the particular interests of the individual.

Any procedure that involves risks to a patient requires contingency plans for resolving complications. The performing radiologist must be prepared to treat such complications or arrange for someone else to assume the responsibility, and this information must be carefully communicated to the patient. At times, this may merely require that the patient be told to contact his or her treating physician immediately if there is a complication (such as clearly described signs of postprocedure infection), or alternatively to go to an emergency room or urgent care center. Failure to attend to this requirement could expose the radiologist to the separate civil tort of *abandonment*.[17]

Some interventional studies may require the radiologist to employ a technique other than that originally planned. For example, if the femoral artery cannot be successfully catheterized for arteriography due to extensive atherosclerotic disease, it may be necessary for the radiologist to use the axillary approach. If the likelihood of using an axillary approach is high, based on the age and symptoms of the patient, the radiologist should include a description of this procedure and its specific complications in the initial consent process. This disclosure must be done expressly, since consent to an arteriogram to be performed in a given manner does not imply consent to an alternate approach with a different spectrum of complications. If no prior consent for an alternative approach has been obtained and the procedure cannot be performed in the expected manner, the radiologist may not then be able to get valid informed consent for the alternative approach because the patient is sedated and not sufficiently awake and alert to assess the different set of potential complications.[18]

Despite intense professional debate, some courts are now requiring physicians to disclose certain information about themselves. This could include underlying medical conditions, such as substance abuse or HIV-positive status, as well as the degree of experience or competence of the radiologist with the proposed procedure.[19]

Withdrawal/Refusal of Consent

A competent patient has the right to withdraw consent at any time and for any reason. Once the patient demands that the radiologist stop a procedure for which consent had been granted, the radiologist must comply with this request and terminate the procedure as soon as it is medically safe to do so.

Occasionally, competent patients may refuse medical treatment necessary to save their lives because of religious or ethical considerations. "If the refusal of medical treatment is truly an informed decision and one that is documented in the medical record ... the radiologist should be protected in the event that a malpractice lawsuit arises from the consequences of the refusal."[20]

Causation

Causation is the most difficult element to prove in informed consent cases.[21] These suits do not allege that a procedure was performed in a negligent manner, but rather that had there been full disclosure of the material risks or available alternatives, the patient would not have undergone the procedure and thus would not have been injured (the "but for" rule). Therefore, the patient must prove that the lack of informed consent (failure to receive sufficient information) was the cause of the injury.[22]

The courts have established two standards of causation. The *objective* standard asks whether a *reasonable person* in the patient's position would have refused consent if properly informed of the potential risks and the possible alternatives. The *subjective* standard determines whether that *specific patient* (not necessarily a "reasonably prudent person" in the patient's position) would have refused to consent if provided with all material information about the procedure. Both of these standards provide substantial protection for the conscientious physician who discloses major risks and then has a more unlikely complication occur. "A patient who consents to a procedure knowing of the risk of death and paralysis will find it difficult to convince a court that knowledge of a minor risk would have led to refusal." A few jurisdictions do not require proof of causation in informed consent cases, effectively considering them as batteries rather than negligence actions.[23]

Exceptions to the Disclosure Requirement

There are four generally recognized exceptions to the physician's duty to make a prior disclosure of material risks, though not all are available in every state. Consent is implied in an emergency in which the patient is unconscious or otherwise incapable of giving valid consent, and the imminent harm from failure to perform a diagnostic or therapeutic procedure outweighs its underlying risks. The physician must document the existence of an actual emergency, that the procedure was for the patient's benefit, and the inability to obtain the express consent of the patient or someone authorized to consent on his or her behalf.[24]

Most courts recognize a "therapeutic privilege," which permits a physician to withhold medical facts from a patient because of the reasonable belief that disclosure would be detrimental by alarming the patient to such a degree that he or she would refuse a necessary diagnostic or therapeutic procedure. However, this requires that the physician can document that the anxiety of the patient is significantly above the norm. In many states, the material information about the risks must be disclosed to a relative, who has to agree with the patient's consent before the procedure may be performed.[25]

The physician does not have to disclose risks that are common knowledge or that the patient has previously experienced or already knows. In addition, a competent patient may waive the right to informed consent by specifically asking not to receive any information about the procedure. However, since courts tend to be skeptical about such waivers, the radiologist should encourage reluctant patients to be fully informed.[26]

In the infrequent circumstances in which informed consent is not obtained because of one of the above situations, the radiologist should carefully document in detail the specific reasons for the omission.

Who Must Disclose?

The radiologist who is to perform the procedure has the responsibility for obtaining consent. The courts have ruled that securing consent is not the duty of a referring physician for procedures ordered or performed by a specialist.[27] A radiologist may delegate the authority to secure consent to another physician, but remains ultimately responsible for having a proper informed consent obtained.[28] If a patient clearly requests that a specific radiologist not perform a procedure and the forbidden radiologist performs it, both the prohibited radiologist and those who permit him or her to perform the procedure can be liable.

Documentation

Although informed consent is a process in which an exchange of information between the physician and patient culminates in the patient's accepting a specific procedure or treatment, it nevertheless is essential that the radiologist document that informed consent was granted. This generally entails the patient's signing a printed consent form and the radiologist's writing a note in the patient's medical record detailing that a discussion regarding informed consent took place.

It is far preferable to employ a customized consent form that contains information unique to the procedure, rather than a generic, hospital-wide form.[29] The consent form should state the name and a description of the specific procedure as well as that (a) the person signing has been told about the radiologic procedure and its risks, benefits, and alternatives; (b) all questions have been answered to the patient's satisfaction; and (c) no guarantees have been made.[30]

A properly signed consent form is strong evidence against any subsequent claim that the patient was uninformed, but it is not conclusive. A person challenging the adequacy of the consent process usually has an opportunity to convince the court that truly informed consent was not actually obtained. One possible challenge is lack of capacity due to transient impairment by medication. Therefore, in nonemergent situations, consent should be obtained before a patient is premedicated for a procedure. A patient may claim that the consent form was too technical and at a too-high level of reading ability. Thus, the consent form should be written so that the person signing can understand it. "Forms in other languages are not required, but they may be useful when a substantial portion of the patients served by the hospital or clinic speak a primary language other than English." If the patient has difficulty understanding English, a translator must be provided. The translator should certify on the document that the consent form and radiologist explanation have been orally translated for the person signing the form. For deaf patients, it may be necessary to provide sign language interpreters.[31] Other challenges to the quality of the consent process include (a) a hostile, antagonistic, pontifical, or condescending manner of the physician obtaining the consent; (b) emotional distress on the part of the patient during the consent process; and (c) lack of time for contemplation and consultation by the patient between the explanation of the risks and benefits of the procedure and being asked to sign the consent form.[32]

Some radiologists have supplemented their explanations with educational materials such as booklets and videotapes. Another approach is to make an audio or video recording of the consent process to supplement or substitute for written consent. Some patients are given tests of knowledge about the proposed procedure or write their own consent forms to document their level of understanding. Although these steps are not legally required and may not preclude malpractice lawsuits, they should be given serious consideration for high-risk procedures.[33]

Endnotes

1 *Schloendorff v New York Hospital*, 105 N.E. 92 (1914).
2 Consent to and refusal of medical treatment. In: Sanbar SS, Gibofsky A, Firestone MH, et al (eds). *Legal Medicine, 5th ed.* St. Louis, Mosby, 2001, pg 246.
3 Miller RD, Hutton RC. *Problems in Health Care Law, 8th ed.* Gaithersburg (MD), Aspen, 2000, pg. 451.
4 Ibid., 452.
5 *Canterbury v Spence*, 464 F2d 772 (DC Cir 1972).
6 Miller RD, Hutton RC. *Problems in Health Care Law, 8th ed.* Gaithersburg (MD), Aspen, 2000, pg. 452.
7 Berlin L. Informed consent. *AJR* 1997;169:15–19.
8 Smith JJ. Intravenous contrast agents: adverse reactions. In: *Risk Management: Test and Syllabus.* Reston, VA: American College of Radiology, 1999:79–87.
9 *Canterbury v Spence*, 464 F2d 772 (DC Cir 1972).
10 Consent to and refusal of medical treatment. In: Sanbar SS, Gibofsky A, Firestone MH, et al (eds). *Legal Medicine, 5th ed.* St. Louis, Mosby, 2001, pg 256.
11 *Keel v St. Elizabeth Medical Center*, 842 S.W.2d 860 (KY 1992).
12 Smith JJ. Intravenous contrast agents: adverse reactions. In: *Risk Management: Test and Syllabus.* Reston, VA: American College of Radiology, 1999:79–87.
13 *Medical-Legal Issues for Residents in Radiology.* Reston, VA: American College of Radiology, 1994:26.
14 *Arato v Avedon*, 5 Cal 4th 1172, 23 Cal Rptr 2d 131, 858 P.2d 298 (1993).
15 Miller RD, Hutton RC. *Problems in Health Care Law, 8th ed.* Gaithersburg (MD), Aspen, 2000, pg. 452–453.
16 Smith JJ. Intravenous contrast agents: adverse reactions. In: *Risk Management: Test and Syllabus.* Reston, VA: American College of Radiology, 1999:79–87.
17 Brenner RJ. Breast interventional procedures. In: *Risk Management: Test and Syllabus.* Reston, VA: American College of Radiology, 1999: 21–27.
18 Ibid.
19 Miller RD, Hutton RC. *Problems in Health Care Law, 8th ed.* Gaithersburg (MD), Aspen, 2000, pg. 453.
20 *Medical-Legal Issues for Residents in Radiology.* Reston, VA: American College of Radiology, 1994:28.
21 Miller RD, Hutton RC. *Problems in Health Care Law, 8th ed.* Gaithersburg (MD), Aspen, 2000, pg. 454.
22 Consent to and refusal of medical treatment. In: Sanbar SS, Gibofsky A, Firestone MH, et al (eds). *Legal Medicine, 5th ed.* St. Louis, Mosby, 2001, pg 256.

23 Miller RD, Hutton RC. *Problems in Health Care Law, 8th ed*. Gaithersburg (MD), Aspen, 2000, pg. 454–455.

24 Consent to and refusal of medical treatment. In: Sanbar SS, Gibofsky A, Firestone MH, et al (eds). *Legal Medicine, 5th ed*. St. Louis, Mosby, 2001, pg 255.

25 Miller RD, Hutton RC. *Problems in Health Care Law, 8th ed*. Gaithersburg (MD), Aspen, 2000, pg. 455.

26 Ibid.

27 Ibid., 456.

28 Consent to and refusal of medical treatment. In: Sanbar SS, Gibofsky A, Firestone MH, et al (eds). *Legal Medicine, 5th ed*. St. Louis, Mosby, 2001, pg 252.

29 Berlin L. Informed consent. *AJR* 1997;169:15–19.

30 Miller RD, Hutton RC. *Problems in Health Care Law, 8th ed*. Gaithersburg (MD), Aspen, 2000, pg. 459.

31 Ibid., 460.

32 Consent to and refusal of medical treatment. In: Sanbar SS, Gibofsky A, Firestone MH, et al (eds). *Legal Medicine, 5th ed*. St. Louis, Mosby, 2001, pg 258.

33 Miller RD, Hutton RC. *Problems in Health Care Law, 8th ed*. Gaithersburg (MD), Aspen, 2000, pg. 462.

22
Do Not Resuscitate (DNR) Orders

As with the right to refuse other unwanted medical treatment, con-stitutional support for the right of an individual to reject unwanted re-suscitation is derived from the "right to privacy" and from the liberty interest protected by the Fourteenth Amendment.[1] National concern with well-publicized legal cases centering on patient self-determination relative to life-preserving treatment and resuscitation, such as those involving Karen Ann Quinlan (1976) and Nancy Cruzan (1990), led to congressional passage of the Patient Self-Determination Act of 1990,[2] which mandates that all institutions receiving Medicare or Med-icaid funds inform all patients of their right to execute an advance care directive.[3] The Joint Commission on Accreditation of Healthcare Organizations has included a similar requirement as one of its stan-dards.[4] Similar guidelines for appropriate use of DNR orders are expressed in the 1991 Code of Medical Ethics of the American Medi-cal Association.[5]

Currently, most hospitals have policies that all patients will be resus-citated, regardless of age or medical condition, unless a written DNR order has been entered in their chart. "As the number of elderly pa-tients entering the health care system increases, and as these individu-als become more active and empowered both legislatively and judicially in assessing and controlling the medical care given them," radiologists increasingly will be placed in situations in which they must decide whether to perform cardiopulmonary resuscitation (CPR). The "reflex resuscitation" of anyone experiencing an arrest, despite the presence of a DNR order, may lead to the institution of a malpractice suit or disciplinary proceedings against the radiologist.[6]

It is usually the responsibility of the primary care physician to discuss the issue of advance directives to determine the patient's deci-sion whether resuscitation should be attempted. "Many attending physicians write DNR orders for patients who are terminally ill and for whom resuscitation would be medically futile or, on balance, would not correspond to the patient's established treatment plan and objectives (e.g., maximal comfort without undue prolongation of life)." In older patients with chronic but nonterminal conditions, such as severe diabetes or arthritis, a DNR order may not reflect medical futility but rather the patient's desire to "die with dignity." Many patients may agree to DNR orders because they fear the complications that may be associated with resuscitation, such as the need for prolonged ventilator support. Others believe that "cardiac arrest, regardless of its cause, is a divine signal that their 'time is up' and that they should die a natural death."[7]

Compliance with DNR Orders

Despite the legislative, regulatory, and ethical guidelines that patients should be given the option of rejecting resuscitation, many physicians remain reluctant to comply with patients' DNR wishes and are convinced that they should respond vigorously to all procedure-related complications. In one study,[8] 60% of anesthesiologists "assumed" that active DNR orders were suspended during the perioperative period; only half discussed this assumption with the patient or guardian, because of lack of experience and confidence in dealing with such a sensitive issue. Most surgeons also feel responsible for treating every procedure-related cardiopulmonary arrest despite the presence of a DNR order,[9] fearing that withholding CPR in such circumstances is tantamount to killing the patient and would expose the surgeon to a malpractice lawsuit for failing to take action in a life-threatening situation.[10]

Radiologists have expressed a variety of reasons for overriding valid DNR orders. Some argue that patients would make different decisions concerning DNR orders if they understood the differences between the radiology suite and the rest of the hospital. In the radiology department some causes of cardiac arrest, such as idiosyncratic reactions to procedures or injections of contrast material, may be treated much more effectively than most primary care physicians or patients would expect. In essence, these radiologists maintain that there is a critical difference between a cardiopulmonary arrest that occurs as the "inevitable, final, and even 'anticipated' outcome of a disease process," in which a DNR order should be honored, and a procedure-related arrest for which radiologists are responsible and for which the patient would want them to attempt resuscitation. Other radiologists note that even if DNR orders are "technically applicable according to policy, guilt and a sense of obligation may lead them to ignore the orders." This is related to a "fear of allegations by patients' families of medical negligence" or the reactions of colleagues accusing them of abandoning their patients in times of need.[11]

Recommended Approach

According to Berlin,[12] "Radiologists should apprise themselves of a patient's DNR status *before* performing any diagnostic or therapeutic radiologic procedure that could reasonably be expected to cause a complication that would require CPR." If the patient is competent, the radiologist (or designee) should initiate a preprocedural discussion with the patient about possible complications and determine whether the patient "wishes to continue or suspend the DNR order while undergoing the procedure." If the patient is incompetent, the discussion should be held with the patient's family or guardian; if neither party is available, the attending physician should be consulted. The radiologist should provide "the likelihood that resuscitative measures would have to be undertaken, a description of the resuscitative techniques that would be applied, an estimate of the chances of success of the resuscitation, and an expected outcome if resuscitation were or were not carried out." All discussions between the radiologist and the patient (or representative) relating to continuing or suspending the DNR order should be precisely documented in the patient's hospital or medical record. If there is any residual doubt about the validity or appropriateness of the DNR order, but no one available to reconsider it, the radiologist should consider postponing the procedure until there is a responsible party with whom to discuss the situation.

Radiologists who clearly discuss resuscitation status with patients before initiating a procedure can avoid the emotional strain and discomfort of suddenly having to decide in a crisis situation whether to honor a DNR order.[13] A radiologist who decides, "after much soul-searching, that it would be unethical to withhold resuscitative efforts for a particular patient" who insists on maintaining the DNR order during the procedure "has no moral obligation to accede to the patient's request if it would conflict with his or her perception of professional obligation." In such cases, the radiologist should "inform the primary physician of the patient's reluctance to forgo the DNR order and, if requested, to aid in finding another radiologist who would be willing to perform the procedure while at the same time respecting the patient's wishes."[14]

Consequences of Failure to Comply with a DNR Order

Despite their good intentions, radiologists who fail to comply with valid DNR orders may be accused of negligence or battery (the intentional touching of another without express or implied consent) by resuscitating the patient against the documented wishes of the patient and his or her family. This potentially could result in a radiologist being held liable for damages for the patient's pain, suffering, disability, and medical expenses incurred during the period from the successful resuscitation to the patient's death. In addition, a radiologist who provides unwanted life-saving treatment in violation of a DNR order may be exposed to disciplinary sanctions by state licensing agencies. Therefore, "radiologists whose conscience or ethical values preclude them from complying with DNR orders should withdraw from the case and respectfully defer to another colleague."[15]

Endnotes

1 The process of dying. In: Sanbar SS, Gibofsky A, Firestone MH, et al (eds). *Legal Medicine, 5th ed.* St. Louis, Mosby, 2001, pg 341.

2 Omnibus Duget Reconciliation Act of 1990. Title IV, Section 4206. Congressional Record. October 26, 1990;136:H12,456–12,457.

3 Berlin, L. Do not resuscitate. *AJR* 2000;175:1513–1517.

4 Joint Commission on Accreditation of Healthcare Organizations. *Standards. R1.1.2.4-1.2.5, Patient Rights and Organization Ethics.* Oakbrook Terrace, IL: Joint Commission on Accreditation of Healthcare Organizations, 2000.

5 American Medical Association Council on Ethical and Judicial Affairs. *Code of Medical Ethics. 2.22. Do-Not-Resuscitate Orders.* Chicago: American Medical Association, 1997:59–61.

6 Berlin L. Do not resuscitate. *AJR* 2000;175:1513–1517.

7 Jacobson JA, Gully JE, Mann H. "Do not resuscitate" orders in the radiology department: an interpretation. *Radiology* 1996;198:21–24.

8 Clemency MV, Thompson NJ. Do not resuscitate (DNR) orders and the anesthesiologist: a survey. *Anesth Analg* 1993;76:394–401.

9 Cohen CB, Cohen PJ. Do-not-resuscitate orders in the operating room. *N Engl J Med* 1991;325:1879–1882.

10 Berlin L. Do not resuscitate. *AJR* 2000;175:1513–1517.

11 Jacobson JA, Gully JE, Mann H. "Do not resuscitate" orders in the radiology department: an interpretation. *Radiology* 1996;198:21–24.

12 Berlin L. Do not resuscitate. *AJR* 2000;175:1513–1517.

13 Jacobson JA, Gully JE, Mann H. "Do not resuscitate" orders in the radiology department: an interpretation. *Radiology* 1996;198:21–24.

14 Terry PB. Resuscitation and radiology. *Radiology* 1996;198:17–18.
15 Berlin L. Do not resuscitate. *AJR* 2000;175:1513–1517.

23
Barium Enema

Perforation of the colon secondary to a barium enema examination is a relatively common cause of malpractice litigation since it often leads to prolonged hospitalization or even death. When a patient complains of acute severe pain (more than the normal fullness or discomfort) during the procedure, the radiologist should not continue unless he or she can exclude the possibility of colonic perforation by showing that there is no extravasation of barium. The increase in hydrostatic pressure associated with a barium enema, especially in a patient with inflammatory disease of the colon, can lead to colonic perforation even if the procedure is performed with meticulous care. When the study is performed by a specially trained technologist or physician assistant, the radiologist may be judged negligent for failure to be physically present during the procedure to monitor the flow of barium fluoroscopically so as to promptly recognize the extravasation of barium and stop the procedure. Technologists taking postprocedure overhead films should be instructed to recognize the clinical signs and symptoms indicating colonic perforation, and the radiologist should be immediately available if this complication becomes evident. The radiologist must be sensitive to the possibility of colonic perforation if the patient experiences acute pain during or following the procedure and be able to detect extravasation of barium on overhead or postprocedure abdominal films, since any delay in treatment may substantially decrease the patient's chance for a successful recovery. If colonic perforation is noted, the radiologist should immediately inform the referring physician and recommend a surgical consultation.[1]

Perforation of the rectum with extravasation of barium secondary to the improper insertion or inflation of a rectal balloon catheter can lead to a malpractice lawsuit. There is controversy within the radiologic community concerning the procedure for inserting enema tips and inflating retention balloons. Some authorities recommend that the radiologist first perform a digital rectal examination to determine whether a retention balloon is necessary and, if so, that the rectal balloon be inflated only by the radiologist (or under the direct supervision of the radiologist).[2] Others disagree, arguing that there is no need for a preliminary rectal examination and that it is acceptable for well-trained technologists to insert enema tips.[3] The American College of Radiology standard states that the enema tip should be inserted by a physician or trained assistant (technologist, nurse, or physician assistant). If a retention cuff is to be used, it "should be inserted carefully.... A physician should be in the fluoroscopic area during cuff insertion."[4] The consensus appears to be that the radiologist should decide whether to use a retention balloon, but may delegate the actual insertion and inflation to an experienced radiologic technologist or nurse.[5]

Courts have rendered divergent opinions as to the liability of a radiologist who was not in the room when a patient's rectum was perforated during tip insertion by a hospital radiologic technologist. One[6] ruled that the radiologist was not vicariously liable, since "nothing in the law required radiologists to be physically present to supervise every activity that takes place in the radiology department."[7] Another[8] took the opposite tack, holding that a patient could sue the radiologist under the doctrine of *res ipsa loquitur* (see page 14), which permits the jury to infer negligent conduct when the adverse event is one that ordinarily does not occur in the absence of negligence.

Endnotes

1 Berlin L. Perforation of the colon during barium enema examination. *AJR* 1996;167:843–845.

2 Barloon TJ, Shumway J. Medical malpractice involving radiologic colon examinations: a review of 38 recent cases. *AJR* 1995;165:343–346.

3 Gelfand DW. Medical malpractice involving barium enema examinations. *AJR* 1995;165:347–348.

4 American College of Radiology. *Standard for the Performance of the Adult Barium Enema Examination*. Reston VA: American College of Radiology, 1995.

5 Berlin L. Perforation of the colon during barium enema examination. *AJR* 1996;167:843–845.

6 *Oberzan v Smith*, 869 P2d 682 (Kan 1994).

7 Berlin L. Perforation of the colon during barium enema examination. *AJR* 1996;167:843–845.

8 *Cassaday v Hendrickson*, 486 NE2d 1329 (Ill App 1985).

24
Breast Imaging

The allegation of error in the diagnosis of breast cancer has become the most common cause of medical malpractice lawsuits against all physicians, with radiologists now the specialists most frequently sued in cases related to this condition. Moreover, mammography has become the most common imaging procedure involved in malpractice suits filed against radiologists.[1,2] As the number of mammographic examinations performed annually in the United States rises, it is likely that there will be a concomitant rise in the number of related malpractice actions.[3] According to one astute observer, the increase in breast cancer litigation (and growing financial awards) are due in great party to the public's misperceptions that (a) women are at extraordinarily high risk of developing and dying from breast cancer; (b) mammography is virtually 100% accurate in revealing early breast cancer; and (c) detecting breast cancer at an early stage guarantees that the malignancy will be cured.[4] In effect, "mammography has been successfully promoted as the best, if not the only, means of detecting breast cancer early and effecting an improved cure rate." Although this has had the positive effect of increasing the number of women undergoing mammograms, it may have also made it extremely difficult for defendant radiologists to prevail in malpractice actions alleging that they failed to detect breast cancer on mammography.[5] As one English radiologist has suggested, many women (and potential jurors of both sexes) falsely believe that screening prevents cancer rather than detects it earlier, that cancers arising after a screening examination with normal findings must have been missed, and that delays in diagnosis inevitably have an adverse effect on the prognosis ("loss of chance" doctrine).[6]

Risk of Women Developing Breast Cancer

The American Cancer Society has sponsored an extremely effective advertising campaign that has led to general public acceptance of the concept that one out of every eight women at any age and at any time will develop breast cancer. In reality, this "one-in-eight" statistic refers to the *cumulative* lifetime risk in women who live past age 85.[7] According to one major study,[8] although breast cancer is already the most common malignancy among women in North America and appears to be further increasing in incidence, the risk of occurrence in a given woman in any specific decade of life never approaches one in eight. A woman entering her 30s has a 1-in-250 chance of developing breast cancer in the next ten years, and a woman entering her 40s has a 1-in-77 chance of developing the disease in the following decade. Although breast cancer is more common in older women, the risk of this malignancy developing in any decade of life never exceeds one in 34. Nevertheless, the major media still carry advertisements stressing the misleading one-in-eight statistic.[9]

Mortality Rates

Breast cancer is generally viewed as the disease women fear most,[10] probably based on a misperception of the true mortality rates. Studies have shown that about 80% of women in whom breast cancer is diagnosed do not die of the disease.[11] At any age, the leading cause of death among women is always something other than breast cancer. Overall, cancer accounts for about 30% of deaths in women, with breast cancer representing only about 20% of fatal malignancies.[12] Never-theless, one survey[13] indicated that "women overestimated their probability of dying of breast cancer by more than 20-fold and the value of screening mammography of reducing that risk by 100-fold"—misper-ceptions that the authors attributed to widespread efforts to promote screening mammography that were accomplished at the cost of creating unnecessary public anxiety through manipulation of data.[14]

Accuracy of Mammography

Numerous advertisements have appeared using dots to compare the average size of tumors detected by regular physician- or self-examination with those revealed by screening mammography, with the latter as small as 1 to 2 mm. This has fostered the unrealistic expectation among the public that mammography is perfect, and the corollary that any failure of the radiologist to detect a minute malignancy must reflect negligence. In reality, in as many as 75% of cases, breast cancers detected at follow-up mammography are visible in retrospect on initial mammograms that were interpreted by competent radiologists as showing normal findings. Therefore, "failure to detect a retrospectively visible abnormality on a screening mammogram is not necessarily negligent, and retrospective reviews do not reflect everyday practice of screening mammography."[15] Multiple studies have reported that about 25% of cancers were missed on mammography.[16,17] Among the reasons that have been suggested as causes for this lack of accuracy are "differences in visual perception ('I just didn't see it'), differences in diagnostic criteria (one interpreting radiologist saying, 'Any calcification may be malignant,' another saying, 'If punctate, calcifications may be benign'), and varying thresholds of concern [for recommending biopsy]".[18] From 5% to 9% of palpable breast cancers are not revealed on mammograms; when cancers that reach clinical detectability within one year after mammography are included, the number increases by 20%.[19] A prominent mammographer has observed that "mammography is not an accurate test because there is considerable overlap in the appearances of benign and malignant lesions on mammograms," emphasizing that "even the most expert doctor will occasionally overlook an important abnormality."[20]

Experienced radiologists disagree among themselves in recommending biopsy versus follow-up about one third of the time when interpreting screening mammograms, and almost half the time when reading diagnostic mammograms.[21] Indeed, the miss and disagreement rates in mammography are so high that there have been numerous suggestions for improving them, such as double reading by a second radiologist,[22] computer-aided detection,[23] and mandating that an individual radiologist interpreting mammograms read a minimum of 2000 annually.[24] Many radiology practices limit the interpreting of mammograms to a few individuals, who devote all or at least most of their time at this task. Radiologists specializing in mammography have been shown to detect more cancers and more early-stage cancers, recommend more biopsies, and have lower recall rates than general radiologists.[25] However, limiting mammography reading to specialists is impractical in many groups and does not represent the standard of care. Attendance at continuing medical education seminars on breast cancer increases the overall accuracy of mammographic interpretations, as does comparing current mammograms with previous studies.[26]

Effect of Mammography on Lengthening Survival Time and Reducing Death Rates

The most contentious issue in breast imaging is whether screening mammography is effective in reducing breast cancer mortality. Based on "statistically significant reductions in breast cancer deaths," the American Cancer Society, the American College of Radiology, and the American Medical Association all recommend annual screening for women beginning at 40 years old; the National Cancer Institute advises screening mammography every 1 to 2 years.[27] However, several researchers have questioned the validity of the conclusion that mammography lowers the mortality rates for breast cancer. The authors of an early article[28] suggested that the increase in breast carcinoma revealed by mammography, as well as the apparent improvement in survival rates, is primarily due to the detection of more ductal carcinoma in situ (DCIS) tumors. Many (or most) of these slow-growing in situ cancers never become large enough to be detected by palpation or to pose a threat to life. They cited prior studies indicating that "small foci of breast cancer are found at autopsy in 39% of women between ages 40 and 50 who died of other causes, most of these tumors never becoming clinically apparent, much less fatal."[29] Moreover, they claimed that the survival rates are misleading due to the statistical phenomena of lead-time and length bias. *Lead-time bias* refers to the fact that pushing back the time of the initial diagnosis by screening mammography merely increases the interval between diagnosis and death, resulting in an apparent but not real lengthening of survival. *Length bias* relates to the fact that more aggressive, rapidly growing malignancies are often found clinically rather than by screening mammography, which primarily detects those that are slower growing and often less dangerous, thus giving the mistaken impression of longer survival.[30]

Subsequent reports have championed or denigrated the effectiveness of screening mammography, and the controversy still rages. Although it seems logical to believe studies that show a reduction in mortality rates from breast cancer in women who have undergone screening mammography, it is extremely difficult to quantify the degree of that decrease and to determine the individual contributions of the various possible causes.[31]

Effect of Delayed Diagnosis of Breast Cancer

A major issue in malpractice lawsuits alleging failure to diagnose breast cancer in a timely fashion is the legal question of proximate cause—the extent to which (if at all) a delayed diagnosis adversely affects treatment and prognosis. Researchers have reported widely divergent views on this topic. One author noted that question of whether early diagnosis reduces mortality from breast cancer remains "one of the most disputed issues in preventive medicine." He pointed out that detecting breast tumors a few months earlier "may make very little difference in their response to treatment," emphasizing the sobering thought that "if tumors are aggressive enough to spread out of the breast, markedly reducing chances of survival, they are likely to have done so already.... In fact, early detection of these tumors may only increase the length of time a woman has to live with a diagnosis of cancer without actually changing her prognosis."[32]

While there is substantial evidence in the radiology literature that a delay in the diagnosis of breast cancer may not necessarily diminish the patient's chance of survival or reduce the patient's chance for cure, these statistical studies may carry little weight with jurors presented with a particular woman with breast cancer that allegedly could have been diagnosed some months or years earlier. Many people are convinced that breast cancer spreads so quickly that even a few months delay in diagnosis will inevitably have dire consequences.[33]

One court[34] has even awarded damages for emotional distress related to a failure to diagnose breast cancer three months earlier. In most contexts, compensation for emotional injury or pain (mental anguish) requires demonstration that the plaintiff has sustained an objective physical injury or the need for additional treatment or loss of chance for survival. In this case, no testimony regarding additional treatment or decreased prognosis was offered at trial; the court held that a reasonable "fear of an increased risk of recurrence of cancer" was sufficient to hold the physician liable for damages.[35]

Screening Versus Diagnostic Mammograms

The American College of Radiology standards define a *screening* mammogram as a "radiological examination to detect unsuspected breast cancer at an early stage in asymptomatic women."[36] A *diagnostic* mammogram "is intended to provide specific analytic evaluation of patients with clinically detected or screening-detected abnormalities."[37]

All mammographic studies should be defined as either screening or as diagnostic breast evaluations. The latter requires on-site monitoring by a radiologist to properly tailor the examination to the needs of the specific patient. If such monitoring was not practical and led to an incomplete evaluation, the patient should be recalled for additional views when a radiologist is to be present.[38]

As Brenner and Berlin noted, "To be properly defined, mammographic masses must be visualized in two orthogonal planes. Reasonable attempts must be made to pinpoint the specific location of a lesion on the mammogram for correlation with physical findings such as a palpable lump or for undertaking further imaging evaluation such as a sonographic or stereotactic biopsy.... When a lesion cannot be sufficiently located, that information should be communicated in the radiologist's report." If there is a palpable abnormality, the radiologist is responsible for determining whether it corresponds to the mammographically evident lesion.[39]

Radiology facilities must have a system in place to ensure that the radiologist interpreting mammography is provided by either the patient or referring physician with information about the patient's medical history and relevant signs and symptoms (such as a palpable mass, skin lesion, or nipple discharge). This written communication may be in the form of a requisition filled out by or for the referring physician, or as a questionnaire filled out by the technologist or the patient. The patient information form should contain a direct question addressing the patient's understanding of why the mammogram is being obtained. This will prevent the patient from later claiming that the only reason she underwent mammography was to evaluate a lump she felt in her breast, while the technologist maintains that the patient told her that the mammogram was routine. (In the absence of written documentation, juries tend to be more sympathetic to the injured patient's recollection of what transpired.) If the technologist fills out the form, the patient should be requested to sign the document to indicate that she has read it and agrees that it is accurate.[40]

The radiologist should not render an interpretation on a mammogram if such clinical information is not available. Even if the absence of clinical information is the fault of the referring physician not providing it or the technologist not having the patient fill out a questionnaire, this does not relieve the radiologist of liability for not knowing whether the patient has "expressed or demonstrated any of the indications that would mandate obtaining a diagnostic rather than a screening mammogram."[41]

If the patient has undergone a previous mammogram, reasonable efforts must be made to obtain it, especially when a potentially significant abnormality is detected on the new study. Reliance on a written report is not acceptable; previous films are critical so that the radiologist can personally compare both sets of mammograms to determine whether there has been a change in the appearance. Brenner notes, "Because many breast cancers grow slowly, comparison should be performed with studies other than the most recent one to detect changes that might otherwise be too subtle to recognize from year to year." He "routinely compares studies separated by approximately 3 years' difference, with additional studies reviewed from earlier (e.g., for asymmetries) or later (e.g., for interval scarring) examinations as needed."[42]

According to other authors, in many radiology practices the need for high efficiency requiring batch interpretations (due to high volumes of mammograms and low reimbursement rates) "makes it impractical to compare mammograms from more than one previous examination, at least during the initial presentation." Moreover, "preplacement (loading) of mammograms on a film multiviewer usually results, de facto, in images from a single reference examination being viewed." They concluded that "mammograms obtained 1 year previously, when available, should be the ones used as a reference."[43] If the prior mammograms are not immediately available, radiologists should note in their formal reports that it was impossible to compare current findings with previous studies and indicate the steps taken to attempt to retrieve them; if these studies later become available, an addendum report may be issued.[44]

Mammographic Errors

In one large study of malpractice lawsuits,[45] image quality was an issue in about 15% of cases; the interpreting radiologist was uniformly held responsible for poor image quality when the cases went to trial. Unlike most of the breast, in which lesions are identifiable on two projections and permit the radiologist to detect them even if they are overlooked on one view, certain anatomic areas are well evaluated only on a single view. For example, "breast tissue associated with the inferior mammary fold or axillary tail region may only be demonstrated routinely on the mediolateral oblique (MLO) projection." Appropriate characterization of an abnormality often depends on obtaining the proper image. Spot compression magnification films usually require a longer radiographic exposure, which may cause microcalcifications to be blurred or virtually undetectable by the effect of motion. Unless positioned skillfully, a spot compression device may displace a lesion from view, resulting in a diagnostic error. The radiologist must always be wary of the danger of *satisfaction of search,* in which the detection of one abnormality distracts the observer from noticing other significant areas of concern. It is essential to review all breast tissue during each study as a screening exercise, regardless of the purpose of the individual examination and even if a lesion has been detected.[46]

Reporting the Mammographic Study

Most clinicians rely on the radiologic interpretation of mammograms, deeming radiologists to be substantially more proficient in detecting and evaluating breast lesions on imaging studies. Consequently, final impressions in mammography reports should be phrased in unambiguous language. An "indeterminate" reading is sufficient for screening mammography when the radiologist is recalling the patient for additional views. If these prove inconclusive, the limitations of the study should be identified. Deferring to "clinical correlation" in a final report is not acceptable; moreover, it "will not excuse the radiologist from liability for any unreasonable mammographic interpretation or insufficient evaluation of an abnormal finding."[47]

The requirements for communicating the results of mammographic screening examinations have some unique aspects. In most imaging studies, the examination is requested to assess a clinical finding or symptom. Because an abnormality is suspected until proven otherwise, both the patient and the clinician anticipate a radiology report on which to base diagnostic and future therapeutic decisions. In contrast, mammographic screening, "whether requested by a physician or directly by the patient, is performed in asymptomatic women in whom normal findings are expected more than 95% of the time. Neither the patient nor the clinician expects that further studies will be required and therefore may not be unduly concerned if no further action, or even communication, occurs after mammographic screening."[48]

While the radiologist may be obliged to personally communicate any significant finding on any imaging study, more direct communication with the responsible clinician is particularly important in mammographic screening, especially for self-referred women. "The radiologist interpreting mammograms of self-referred patients is deemed to be acting as the primary care physician for the patient and is directly responsible for the patient's care until a documented referral to an appropriate physician, who is willing to accept the care of the patient."[49]

Multiple factors may contribute to delays in communicating mammographic results to referring physicians and self-referred women. Written reports may be sent to the wrong address if referring physicians have more than one office or clinic location from which they may request mammograms. Reports may be misplaced by personnel in the referring physician's office. At times, reports are simply misunderstood by physicians or their assistants, so that follow-up studies are scheduled in 6 months rather than immediately as recommended by the radiologist who interpreted the screening mammogram. Communicating directly with patients may pose a challenge, since some may not have a telephone, speak English, or provide a current address.[50]

Communication problems with referring physicians, as well as the growing number of self-referrals, have led some radiologists to communicate mammography results and recommendations directly to patients. Studies have shown that this can lead to compliance rates approaching 100% for recommendations for additional imaging, follow-up examinations, or biopsies.[51] Furthermore, direct communication with the patient reduces the anxiety associated with waiting for the results of her mammographic examination.[52]

Many radiologists are reluctant to communicate the results of tests directly to patients, based on a variety of factors. These include "the inherent nature and training of radiologists, a lack of time, medicolegal concerns [and] a worry of offending patients' referring physicians." However, the most important reason is probably a fear of the emotional impact on a woman with an unfavorable mammographic result, who presumably would prefer to receive the bad news from a family physician with whom she has already established a rapport. Nevertheless, one study has shown that a majority of women would prefer radiologists to directly give them mammographic results on site, whether they be normal or abnormal. Similarly, most wished that radiologists "would inform them directly of the need for a short-term follow-up examination, send them reminders before the appointment for the recommended follow-up examination, and contact them directly if they fail to comply."[53]

False-Negative Core Biopsy of the Breast

It is estimated that between 500,000 and 1 million breast biopsies are performed annually in the United States, with an increasing percentage of them being done by radiologists using imaging guidance.[54] Although large-core needle biopsy produces a diagnostic yield rate similar to that achieved by surgical excision,[55] radiologists who perform imaging-guided biopsies "face considerably more medical-legal risk than their surgical colleagues who perform open biopsies."[56] Malpractice lawsuits involving percutaneous core biopsies usually involve allegations against the radiologist for (a) lacking proper indications for biopsy; (b) using improper technique in performing it; (c) or inadequately monitoring the patient when the pathologic results were negative for malignant change.[57]

In determining those patients on whom stereotactic and sonographically guided biopsy will be performed, radiologists should use stringent selection criteria, avoiding cases where the mammographic appearance or location make it likely that the biopsy will be unsuccessful or nondiagnostic. For example, lesions close to the chest wall or axilla, or those high in the upper inner quadrant, may be difficult to biopsy under stereotactic guidance even with a prone table, and thus the patient should be referred for an excisional rather than percutaneous core biopsy.[58] The choice of image-guided versus excisional biopsy also will depend on the experience of the radiologist, the type of equipment available, and the philosophy of the attending surgeon. Those who perform one-stage surgical procedures encompassing both diagnosis and treatment generally do not recommend radiologically performed, minimally invasive biopsies for their patients, whereas they are likely to be suggested by those surgeons who prefer a two-stage procedure.[59,60]

Multiple specimens of the lesion should be obtained to decrease the chance of sampling error. One study stressed the importance of taking at least five specimens when biopsying a mass and even more when there are only microcalcifications. It reported that the first specimen of a solid mass yielded a diagnosis in 70% of cases, whereas the yield increased to 99% when five specimens were obtained.[61] Biopsies of the breast generally have a higher percentage of diagnoses when using a 14-gauge needle than a smaller 18-gauge one.[62] Radiologic-pathologic correlation should be performed and documented in every case. If the findings are discordant—with the radiologist performing the core biopsy concluding that the appearance of the mammographic lesion is suggestive of carcinoma despite histologic findings that fail to show malignant changes—an excisional biopsy should be recommended. [63]

Specimen Radiography[64]

Specimen radiography is mandatory following imaging-guided core biopsy to ensure that the region of interest has been biopsied, and after open surgical resection to make certain that a nonpalpable mammographic abnormality has been completely excised. Initially, specimen radiography was considered of value only for calcified lesions to reduce the incidence of false-negative biopsies. However, technical improvements have shown similar accuracy in the radiography of noncalcified lesions. Nevertheless, "certain non-calcified masses, focal asymmetries, architectural distortions, and subtle microcalcifications may be difficult to detect on specimen radiography. Most of these abnormalities will be detected with the use of compression or magnification views." The specimen should be radiographed in two dimensions, promptly correlated with a preoperative mammogram, and interpreted without delay. The radiologist should communicate these findings to the surgeon in the operating room before closure so that additional tissue can be removed if necessary. "In health care facilities in which surgeons or other non-radiologic physicians perform breast biopsies, radiologists should develop and have approved by the administration or the medical executive committee a policy that mandates radiography of all breast biopsy specimens regardless of whether the biopsies are performed in surgery or in the radiology department, whether by radiologists or nonradiologic physicians." This will prevent a situation in which a radiologist may be held liable for the refusal of a surgeon to comply with a radiology department policy that mandates specimen radiography. If the surgeon violates such a policy by refusing to send the biopsy tissue for specimen radiography, the radiologist should recommend in writing that a mammogram be obtained as soon after surgery as the patient can tolerate compression to document the complete removal of a nonpalpable mammographic lesion.

Tracking Patients with Negative Biopsies

Patients who have undergone imaging-guided biopsies should have the same follow-up as women who have had routine screening or diagnostic mammography. The generally accepted practice in the radiology community is to obtain mammography in six months to reassess previously detected mammographic abnormalities that were found to be benign on percutaneous core biopsy. However, if the radiologic and pathologic examinations agree that the lesion is benign, short-term follow-up may not be necessary.[65]

Unfortunately, patients are often lost to follow-up, despite an efficient monitoring system and repeated reminders from the radiology department. This may expose radiologists who interpret mammograms and perform percutaneous biopsies to an ever-increasing risk of malpractice lawsuits. In one study of women who had undergone percutaneous biopsy and received mailed reminder notices and telephone calls from the radiology department, one quarter failed to appear for recommended surgical biopsy and almost half never came in for follow-up surveillance mammography.[66]

This raises the vexing problem of the degree to which radiologists are responsible for tracking patients who have abnormal mammograms or percutaneous biopsies yielding negative findings. The Mammography Quality Standards Act (MQSA) states, "Each facility must have a system to track positive mammographic findings and a process to correlate such findings with the biopsy results the facility has obtained."[67] Similarly, the Agency for Health Care Policy and Research, a division of the United States Department of Health and Human Services, notes that the facility that performed the initial mammography examination should be responsible for performing or arranging for future examinations and any immediate additional views or studies, though it adds that "the referring health care provider is responsible for the follow-up, monitoring, and tracking of women whose results are abnormal."[68] The American College of Radiology states that radiologists should follow up all biopsies to determine "the rate of compliance with the recommended follow-up" and to "detect and record any false-negative or false-positive results."[69]

Unfortunately, none of these publications provides any specific information as to how radiologists should accomplish the required tracking and monitoring of the patient with abnormal findings on mammography or equivocal biopsy results. This is a critical medical-legal issue, since in about 75% of all breast cancer cases in which payments are made, the plaintiff has alleged a lack of appropriate follow-up.[70] It is evident that "radiologists must develop and carefully adhere to a policy that details a tracking and monitoring process," but there is no national or community standard as to what it should contain. The best method (regular or certified mail, telephone calls) and frequency of communication to the patient are unclear. Regardless of the system employed, "radiologists should carefully document in writing every written and verbal reminder for follow-up mammographic examinations communicated to patients." Radiologists cannot physically force a woman to return for a follow-up examination, since patients always retain the right to refuse mammography if they wish. As in other areas of malpractice, radiologists must strive to act in a "reasonable" manner, realizing that the ultimate legal decision as to whether a radiologist's efforts to communicate with the plaintiff were sufficiently aggressive and effective lies in the hands of a jury.[71]

Endnotes

1 Physician Insurers Association of America. *Breast Cancer Study.* Rockville, MD: Physician Insurers Association of America, 1995.

2 Physician Insurers Association of America and American College of Radiology. *Practice Standards Claims Survey*. Rockville, MD: Physician Insurers Association of America, 1997.

3 Berlin L. The missed breast cancer redux: time for educating the public about the limitations of mammography? *AJR* 2001;176:1131–1134.

4 Berlin L. Dot size, lead time, fallibility, and impact on survival: continuing controversies in mammography. *AJR* 2001;176:1123–1130.

5 Berlin L. The missed breast cancer redux: time for educating the public about the limitations of mammography? *AJR* 2001;176:1131–1134.

6 Wilson RM. Screening for breast and cervical cancer as a common cause for litigation. *BMJ* 2000;320:1352–1353.

7 Berlin L. Dot size, lead time, fallibility, and impact on survival: continuing controversies in mammography. *AJR* 2001;176:1123–1130.

8   Phillips KA, Glendon G, Knight JA. Putting the risk of breast cancer in perspective. *N Engl J Med* 1999;340:141–144.

9   *New York Times*, October 3, 2000:C3.

10 Berlin L. Dot size, lead time, fallibility, and impact on survival: continuing controversies in mammography. *AJR* 2001;176:1123–1130.

11 Phillips KA, Glendon G, Knight JA. Putting the risk of breast cancer in perspective. *N Engl J Med* 1999;340:141–144.

12 *Mayo Clinic Update*. Rochester, MN: Mayo Foundation for Medical Education and Research, 1999;15(2):4.

13 Black WC, Nease RF Jr, Tosteson ANA. Perceptions of breast cancer risk and screening effectiveness in women younger than 50 years of age. *J Natl Cancer Inst* 1995;87:721–731.

14 Berlin L. The missed breast cancer. Perceptions and realities. *AJR* 1999;173:1161–1167.

15 Ibid.

16 Georgen SK, Evans J, Cohen GHP, MacMillan JH. Characteristics of breast carcinomas missed by screening radiologists. *Radiology* 1997;204:131–135.

17 Kerlikowshe K, Grady D, Barclay J, et al. Variability and accuracy in mammography interpretation using the American College of Radiology breast imaging reporting and data system. *J Natl Cancer Inst* 1998;90:1801–1809.

18 Berlin L. The missed breast cancer. Perceptions and realities. *AJR* 1999;173:1161–1167.

19 Kopans DB. *Breast Imaging*, 2nd ed. Philadelphia: Lippincott-Raven, 1998:749.

20 Brody JE. Mammogram interpretations are questioned in a report. *New York Times*, December 2, 1994:B1.

21 Berg WA, Campassi C, Langenberg P, Sexton MJ. Breast imaging reporting and data system: inter- and intraobserver variability in feature analysis and final assessment. *AJR* 2000;174:1769–1777.

22 Kopans DB. Double reading. *Radiol Clin North Am* 2000;38:719–724.

23 Burhenne LJW, Wood SA, D'Orsi CJ, et al. Potential contribution of computer-aided detection to the sensitivity of screening mammography. *Radiology* 2000;215:554–562.

24 Kan L, Olivotto IA, Burhenne LJW, et al. Standardized abnormal interpretation and cancer detection ratios to assess reading volume and reader performance in a breast screening program. *Radiology* 2000;215:563–567.

25 Sickles EA, Wolverton DE, Dee KE. Performance parameters for screening and diagnostic mammography: specialist and general radiologists. *Radiology* 2002;224:861–869.

26 Berlin L. The missed breast cancer. Perceptions and realities. *AJR* 1999;173:1161–1167.

27 Feig SA. Age-related accuracy of screening mammography: how should it be measured? *Radiology* 2000;214:633–640.

28 Black WC, Welch HG. Advances in diagnostic imaging and overestimation of disease prevalence and the benefits of therapy. *N Engl J Med* 1993;328:1237–1243.

29 Berlin L. The missed breast cancer. Perceptions and realities. *AJR* 1999; 173:1161–1167.

30 Ibid.

31 Berlin L. Dot size, lead time, fallibility, and impact on survival: continuing controversies in mammography. *AJR* 2001;176:1123–1130.

32 Zuger A. Do breast self-exams save lives? Science still doesn't have the answer. *New York Times*, January 6, 1998:B9,15.

33 Berlin L. The missed breast cancer redux: time for educating the public about the limitations of mammography? *AJR* 2001;176:1131–1134.

34 *Boryla v Pash*, 960 P2d 123 (Colo 1998).

35 Berlin L. The missed breast cancer redux: time for educating the public about the limitations of mammography? *AJR* 2001;176:1131–1134.

36 ACR Standards 2000-2001. *ACR Standard for the Performance of Screening Mammography 2000*. Reston, VA: American College of Radiology, 2000:39–46.

37 ACR Standards 2000-2001. *ACR Standard for the Performance of Diagnostic Mammography 1999*. Reston, VA: American College of Radiology, 2000:47–53.

38 Brenner RJ, Berlin L. Evaluation of the mammographic abnormality. *AJR* 1996;167: 17–19.

39 Ibid.

40 Homer MJ, Berlin L. Mammography and the patient information form. *AJR* 2002;178:307–310.

41 Berlin L. Screening versus diagnostic mammogram. *AJR* 1999;173:3–7.

42 Brenner RJ. False-negative mammograms: medical, legal, and risk management implications. *Radiol Clin North Am* 2000;38:741–757.

43 Sumkin JH, Holbert BL, Herrmann JS, et al. Optimal reference mammography: a comparison of mammograms obtained 1 and 2 years before the present examination. *AJR* 2003;180:343–346.

44 Brenner RJ, Berlin L. Evaluation of the mammographic abnormality. *AJR* 1996;167:17–19.

45 Physician Insurers Association of America and American College of Radiology. *Practice Standards Claims Survey*. Rockville, MD: Physician Insurers Association of America, 1997.

46 Brenner RJ. False-negative mammograms: medical, legal, and risk management implications. *Radiol Clin North Am* 2000;38:741–757.

47 Brenner RJ, Berlin L. Evaluation of the mammographic abnormality. *AJR* 1996;167:17–19.

48 Robertson CL, Kopans DB. Communication problems after mammographic screening. *Radiology* 1989;172:443–444.

49 Ibid.

50 Ibid.

51 Cardenosa G, Eklund GW. Rate of compliance with recommendations for additional mammographic views and biopsies. *Radiology* 1991;181:359–361.

52 Hoffman NY, Janus J, Destounis S, Logan-Young W. When the patient asks for the results of her mammogram, how should the radiologist reply? *AJR* 1994;162:597–599.

53 Liu S, Bassett LW, Sayre J. Women's attitudes about receiving mammographic results directly from radiologists. *Radiology* 1994;193:783–786.

54 Bassett L, Winchester DP, Caplan, RB, et al. Stereotactic core-needle biopsy of the breast: a report of the joint task force of the American College of Radiology, American College of Surgeons and College of American Physicians. *CA Cancer J Clin* 1997;47:171–190.

55 Parker SH, Burbank F, Jackman RJ, et al. Percutaneous large-core breast biopsy: a multi-institutional study. *Radiology* 1994;193:359–364.

56 Recenstein MJ, Berlin L. False-negative core biopsy of the breast. *AJR* 1998;171:927–930.

57 Ibid.

58 Philpotts LE, Lee CH, Horvath LJ, Tocino I. Cancelled stereotactic core-needle biopsy of the breast: analysis of 89 cases. *Radiology* 1997;205:423–428.

59 Gisvold JJ, Goellner JR, Grant CS, et al. Breast biopsy: a comparative study of stereotaxically guided core and excisional techniques. *AJR* 1994;162:815–820.

60 Brenner RJ, Fajardo L, Fisher PR, et al. Percutaneous core biopsy of the breast: effect of operator experience and number of samples on diagnostic accuracy. *AJR* 1996;166:341–346.

61 Liberman L, Dershaw DD, Rosen PP, et al. Stereotaxic 14-gauge breast biopsy: how many core biopsy specimens are needed? *Radiology* 1994;192:793–795.

62 Nath ME, Robinson TM, Tobon H, et al. Automated large-core needle biopsy of surgically removed breast lesions: comparison of samples obtained with 14-, 16-, and 18-gauge needles. *Radiology* 1995;197:739–742.

63 Recenstein MJ, Berlin L. False-negative core biopsy of the breast. *AJR* 1998;171:927–930.

64 Homer MJ, Berlin L. Radiography of the surgical breast biopsy specimen. *AJR* 1998;171:1197–1199.

65 Recenstein MJ, Berlin L. False-negative core biopsy of the breast. *AJR* 1998;171:927–930.

66 Goodman KA, Birdwell RL, Ikeda DM. Compliance with recommended follow-up after percutaneous breast core biopsy. *AJR* 1998;170:89–92.

67 Houn F. *What a Mammography Facility Should Do to Prepare for the MQSA Inspection*. Rockville, MD: Unites States Department of Health and Human Services, Food and Drug Administration, 1994.

68 Bassett LW, Henrik RE, Bassford TL. *High-Quality Mammography: Information for Referring Providers* (Agency for Health Care Policy and

Research no. 95-0633). Rockville, MD: United States Department of Health and Human Services, 1994.

69 American College of Radiology. *ACR Standard for Performance of Stereotactically Guided Breast Interventional Procedures*. Reston, VA: American College of Radiology, 1996.

70 Physician Insurers Association of America and American College of Radiology. *Practice Standards Claims Survey*. Rockville, MD: Physician Insurers Association of America, 1997.

71 Berlin L. Tracking of breast cancer. *AJR* 1998;170:93–95.

25
Interventional Procedures

Even the most routine special procedures, such as arteriography, central venous catheter placement, percutaneous needle biopsy, and catheter drainage, can result in serious injury or death. Because these complications are rare, they often lead to malpractice litigation based on the suspicion that negligence or gross error must have occurred.[1] In one long-term study, up to 20% of all malpractice suits filed against radiologists involved complications of procedures.[2] Because there is inherent risk in any procedure, informed consent (see chapter 21) is mandatory. An appropriate imaging guidance method must be selected based on the circumstances of the case and the experience of the individual radiologist. Blood tests are required to identify patients with coagulation defects or other potential predispositions to bleeding during and following the procedure.[3]

Although a procedural complication may lead to malpractice litigation, this does not automatically imply that the plaintiff will be successful. As one court concluded, "The unfortunate fact that [the patient] died as a result of a complication does not mean that [the doctor] was negligent, even if the risk of death during such an operation is slim.... If a doctor exercised a reasonable degree of care and skill under the circumstances as they existed, and not as we see them in perfect hindsight, then the doctor is not guilty of malpractice.... Medicine is an imperfect science.... Operations of this nature have risks."[4]

Technical Issues

The radiologist must address technical issues related to the specific interventional procedure. For example, before performing a percutaneous needle biopsy it is essential to identify all major blood vessels in the region so that they can be avoided. When the lesion to be biopsied is near a major vessel, it may be advisable to begin with a smaller-gauge needle, and then increase the size of the needle if the initial sample is not adequate.[5] When placing a central venous catheter in the sub-clavian vein, the radiologist should minimize the number of needle passes, which has a positive correlation with the complication rate.[6] When performing an arteriogram, care must be taken to avoid punctur-ing either the iliac or superficial femoral artery, lest an inability to com-press the vessel leads to the development of a large hematoma or pseudoaneurysm.[7] When different approaches are available, the radi-ologist must weigh their potential risks carefully, selecting the one that can accomplish the required goal in the safest manner for the patient.

Interventional radiologists should always remember that "a failed pro-cedure is better than a catastrophe. If the attempted procedure is be-coming substantially more risky to the patient than anticipated, the radiologist should strongly consider stopping and postponing the proce-dure for another day." This allows time to discuss the situation with both the patient and the referring physician, as well as to suggest alter-native approaches that might succeed without unnecessary risks.[8]

The radiologist should carefully document the procedure and keep a complete and accurate medical record, which can be invaluable if a case subsequently becomes the subject of a malpractice lawsuit. This documentation of the order of the steps taken during the procedure and the reasoning behind them is particularly important when nonstandard methods are used.[9] In such cases, the radiologist should be able to describe the advantages (and disadvantages) of any alternative tech-nique, as well as cite supporting articles in the medical literature and presentations by recognized experts at scientific meetings to indicate that the approach selected is employed by not just one or a few radiolo-gists but rather by a respectable number of similarly trained and prac-ticing radiologists (the so-called "two schools of thought" doctrine; see page 12).[10]

Postprocedure Care

Although may radiologists believe that they have completely fulfilled their role once an interventional procedure has ended, "in the eyes of the patient and the law the radiologist has a clear responsibility to par-ticipate actively in post-procedure care, especially in patients in whom complications develop." To detect possible complications, the radiolo-gist should make a postprocedure visit to inpatients and a follow-up telephone call to outpatients.[11] Communication with the patient after (and before) the procedure is an effective deterrent to litigation in the event of an adverse outcome.[12] Despite the natural feelings of many radiologists that they do not possess the same level of bedside skills as their clinical colleagues, they often are the most experienced physicians available to deal with complications of interventional procedures. Consequently, radiologists should have no hesitancy in suggesting possible remediable causes of procedural complications. "Because postprocedure hemorrhage is the most common serious complication, radiologists must have a high index of suspicion when a patient experiences tachycardia, hypotension, or increasing pain ... [and] be aggressive in recommending imaging to detect bleeding." Although CT is highly sensitive for the presence of blood, arteriography may be required to demonstrate the precise site of postprocedure hemorrhage and provide a nonsurgical approach for controlling it.[13]

Of course, the radiologist is primarily responsible for initiating immediate treatment if a complication arises while the patient is still in the imaging department. If a patient may be bleeding, the radiologists must be "prepared to undertake such therapeutic measures as administering high-volume IV fluid and supplemental oxygen, typing and crossmatching the patient's blood for possible transfusion, and ordering the transfer of the patient to an intensive care unit or other department capable of providing the necessary level of care."[14]

Endnotes

1 Spies JB, Berlin L. Complications of central venous catheter placement. *AJR* 1997;169:339–341.
2 Berlin L, Berlin JW. Malpractice and radiologists in Cook County, IL: trends in 20 years of litigation. *AJR* 1995;165:781–788.
3 Spies JB, Berlin L. Complications of percutaneous needle biopsy. *AJR* 1998;171:13–17.
4 *MacGuineas v United States*, 738 F Supp 566 (DC 1990).
5 Spies JB, Berlin L. Complications of percutaneous needle biopsy. *AJR* 1998;171:13–17.
6 Mansfield PR, Hohn DC, Fornage BD, et al. Complications and failures of subclavian-vein catheterization. *N Engl J Med* 1994;331:1735–1738.
7 Spies JB, Berlin L. Complications of femoral artery puncture. *AJR* 1998;170: 9–11.
8 Spies JB, Berlin L. Complications of central venous catheter placement. *AJR* 1997;169:339–341.
9 Ibid.
10 Mueller PR, Berlin L. Complications of lung abscess aspiration and drainage. *AJR* 2002;178:1083–1086.

11 Spies JB, Berlin L. Complications of percutaneous needle biopsy. *AJR* 1998;171:13–17.

12 Spies JB, Berlin L. Complications of central venous catheter placement. *AJR* 1997;169:339–341.

13 Spies JB, Berlin L. Complications of percutaneous needle biopsy. *AJR* 1998;171:13–17.

14 Ibid.

26
Ionic Versus Nonionic Contrast Material

Currently, there are two major categories of iodinated contrast agents—high and low osmolar. With high-osmolar ("ionic") contrast there is a small, but well-recognized, risk of adverse reactions, some of which are life threatening. However, the vast majority of patients receiving high-osmolar contrast do not experience any significant side effects. Low-osmolar ("non-ionic") contrast has a substantially lower rate of serious reactions (though not fatalities), but is considerably more expensive even in view of a significant decrease in price over the past few years.[1]

The large cost difference between ionic and nonionic contrast material, combined with the extremely low risk of a serious adverse reaction with either agent, has led many radiology groups to adopt a selective-use policy. Believing that the universal use of nonionic contrast is prohibitively expensive, they reserve it for patients perceived to be at a high risk for contrast reactions. According to a publication of the American College of Radiology (ACR), those considered at high risk for contrast reaction include patients with "a history of previous adverse reaction to contrast material, with the exception of a sensation of heat, flushing, or a single episode of nausea and vomiting; a history of allergy or asthma; cardiac dysfunction, including recent or potentially imminent cardiac decompensation, severe arrhythmias, unstable angina pectoris, recent myocardial infarction, and pulmonary hypertension; and generalized severe debilitation."[2] Other risk factors that should be considered as possible indications for the use of nonionic contrast include "(1) sickle cell disease; (2) an increased risk of aspiration; (3) great anxiety about the procedure; and (4) an inability to establish sufficient communication to determine the presence of risk factors."[3] Some authorities have recommended that nonionic contrast also be given to patients with diabetes mellitus and those at the extremes of age (very old or very young). Nonionic contrast is also advisable in patients who have an increased likelihood of extravasation[4] or in whom an injection rate greater than

2.5 mL/sec is to be used,[5] since extravascular hyperosmolar contrast can result in severe skin ulceration and necrosis.

Proponents of the universal use of nonionic contrast argue that, since it is impossible to determine in advance those patients who are truly at high risk, all patients should receive the safest contrast available—nonionic agents. They also believe that radiologists who use nonionic contrast agents selectively will be in greater legal jeopardy in the event of a serious complication. This concept is supported by many legal commentators, who note that courts have historically favored the interest of patients and have generally not considered the costs of services in evaluating whether they should be provided. However, in the absence of any published state appellate court decision addressing the contrast material controversy, no one really knows how the courts will deal with this issue.[6]

As part of basic informed consent, patients should be informed of the risk that accompanies every intravenous administration of contrast material. An intriguing question is what the patient should be told about the differences between ionic and nonionic contrast (and any options the patient may have as to which is used) when a selective-use policy is in place. Especially in states following the reasonable-patient standard (see page 141), a strong argument could be made that a reasonable patient being considered for ionic contrast administration would want to know that a safer, albeit more expensive, alternative is available. This may even require that the radiologist offer to provide nonionic contrast on demand, perhaps at the patient's expense if he or she is at low risk for a contrast reaction. However, this raises the disturbing ethical dilemma of creating a double standard for indigent and wealthy patients. Moreover, federal law forbids a physician from receiving payment from a Medicare beneficiary for nonionic contrast if the patient does not meet the Medicare requirements for its use.[7]

From the risk management perspective, each radiology facility should have a written policy that covers all aspects of the use of contrast media: "Whether non-ionic agents are to be administered universally or selectively; who is authorized to perform IV injections (the ACR standard[8] approves injection by licensed radiologic technologists and nurses under the direction of a radiologist); what type, if any, of informed consent must be obtained; what techniques, needles, and catheters are to be used; when and in what settings pressure injectors should be used; and what steps should be taken in case of an adverse reaction." If nonionic contrast is to be injected on a selective basis, it is essential to define the specific indications for its use. Any deviation from this policy should be documented in the patient's radiology report or in a log kept in the radiology facility.[9]

Radiologists should always remember that they are ultimately responsible for discovering potential risk factors, even if not provided by the referring physician or the patient. If the patient is a poor historian, nonionic contrast should be given since the inability to establish the existence of risk factors is itself deemed a factor in classifying the patient as high risk.[10]

Endnotes

1 Smith JJ. Intravenous contrast agents: adverse reactions. In: *Risk Management. Test and Syllabus*. Reston, VA: American College of Radiology, 1999:75–97.

2 Ibid.

3 Ibid.

4 Dunnick NR. Patient outcome from ionic versus nonionic contrast agents (answer to question). *AJR* 1995;164:1547.

5 Hopper KD. Contrast for bolus injections in helical CT (answer to question). *AJR* 1996;166:715.

6 Berlin L. Ionic versus nonionic contrast media. *AJR* 1996;167:1095–1097.

7 Smith JJ. Intravenous contrast agents: adverse reactions. In: *Risk Management. Test and Syllabus*. Reston, VA: American College of Radiology, 1999:75–97.

8 American College of Radiology. *ACR Standard for Excretory Urography*. Reston, VA: American College of Radiology, 1995.

9 Berlin L. Ionic versus nonionic contrast media. *AJR* 1996;167:1095–1097.

10 Smith JJ. Intravenous contrast agents: adverse reactions. In: *Risk Management. Test and Syllabus*. Reston, VA: American College of Radiology, 1999:75–97.

27
Sedation and Analgesia

Sedation and analgesia has replaced the term *conscious sedation* to describe a "clinical state that allows patients to tolerate unpleasant procedures while maintaining adequate cardiorespiratory function and protective reflexes as well as the ability to respond purposefully to verbal command."[1] Although sedation and analgesia are most frequently employed in the pediatric age range, about 20% of sedated patients are adults, who require medication either to overcome claustrophobia related to an MRI examination or as an integral component of an interventional radiologic procedures. According to the Joint Commission on Accreditation of Healthcare Organizations, each institution should establish and implement a uniform sedation policy to be followed in all clinical areas.

Pediatric Patients[2]

Because of reports of deaths in children undergoing sedation, which is frequently employed for diagnostic or therapeutic procedures, the American Academy of Pediatrics (AAP) was the first to draw the attention of the medical community to the need to improve the sedation practices by issuing a series of guidelines in 1985. The American College of Radiology (ACR) adopted a Standard for Pediatric Sedation/Analgesia in 1998, based on the AAP guidelines and those promulgated by the American Society of Anesthesiologists.

"Sedation is a continuum; conscious sedation may progress to deep sedation depending on the absorption of medications, the amount of stimulation, and other factors." In a large study of children who received conscious sedation for orthopedic emergencies, half were unexpectedly deeply sedated during a portion of their care. Inadvertent deep sedation can cause alterations in respiratory status (reduced respiratory rate, decreased oxygen saturation), which must be immediately treated by noninvasive techniques to improve airway patency and oxygenation. Because of the possible need for urgent intervention, the ACR Standard states: "A designated individual, *other than* the practitioner performing the imaging procedure, must be present to monitor the patient throughout the procedures performed with sedation/analgesia. This individual may assist with minor, interruptible tasks." The sedation monitor must be familiar with airway patency techniques (chin-lift, jaw-thrust, verbal breathing reminders) and have training in pediatric basic life support and cardiopulmonary resuscitation. It is recommended that an individual with pediatric advanced life support skills be on site. The drug naloxone should be available for emergency use to reverse opioid-induced hypoxemia or apnea; in addition, supplemental oxygen and positive-pressure ventilation must be easily accessible in case basic treatment for airway obstruction is unsuccessful. Because of the possible need for urgent intervention, an individual can monitor only one sedated patient at a time.

"The most frequent side effects from the commonly used sedative agents are respiratory depression, vomiting, and agitation. Transient hypoxemia, if uncorrected, can lead to respiratory complications." Because cardiac monitoring and clinical observation is not adequate to recognize developing hypoxemia in children, all patients should be monitored by pulse oximetry; "monitoring of heart rate and rhythm, respiratory function, and level of consciousness is also required." Oral intake of clear liquids can continue until 2 hours before the scheduled procedure.

"A child who is undergoing conscious sedation is expected to be able to withdraw from a painful stimulus, such as suturing of a laceration, and say 'ouch.'" Consequently, a local anesthetic may be necessary to control discomfort and decrease movement during a painful procedure. Although there may be a temptation to give additional sedation so that the child does not move, this practice is inappropriate since it does not decrease the level of pain. "Allowing the child to become non-responsive to pain causes a transition from conscious sedation toward deep sedation," which is defined as "a medically controlled state of depressed consciousness or unconsciousness from which the patient is not easily aroused. It may be accompanied by a partial or complete loss of protective reflexive reflexes and includes the inability to maintain a patent airway independently and respond purposefully to physical stimulation or verbal command." In addition to the equipment needed for conscious sedation, deep sedation in a pediatric patient requires the availability of an electrocardiographic monitor and defibrillator, an intravenous line in place (or the immediate availability of a person skilled in establishing intravenous access in children), and close monitoring (evaluation and documentation of patient status every 5 minutes).

Adult Magnetic Resonance Imaging[3]

Patients often experience claustrophobia or anxiety that requires some degree of sedation to successfully complete an MRI examination. Although the radiologist must beware of potential cardiopulmonary and central nervous system complications of sedation, a more practical danger may be the risk of injury if an unaccompanied patient who is still drowsy attempts to drive home after the study. "Malpractice litigation arising from such injuries can involve not only the facility in which the MR imaging was obtained, but also the radiologist and referring physician."

Radiologists must be aware of the time course associated with the level of sedation and analgesia used in MRI. One large study found that patients required 7 to 42 minutes after the administration of the first medication to be sufficiently sedated to undergo the procedure. The duration of sedation varied from 36 to 90 minutes, while the total procedure time from drug administration to the patient's awakening was 1 to 2 hours. More than one quarter of patients required a second sedative dose, because of either inadequate initial sedation or a prolonged examination; 2.6% received a third medication dose. Therefore, some patients treated with sedation and analgesia for an MRI examination will still be under the influence of the medication for a substantial period after the procedure has ended, posing a serious risk to themselves and others if allowed to immediately drive home.

Consequently, radiologists involved in MRI should seriously consider having in place a written policy that details the way in which sedation and analgesia medication are administered to patients, how they will be monitored during the procedure, and when they can be safely discharged. Once a policy is adopted, the facility should scrupulously adhere to it provisions, since "failure to follow even the letter of the written policy may jeopardize the successful defense of a malpractice lawsuit that involves a sedation or post-sedation patient injury." Adult patients requiring sedation should be informed that since they will not be able to drive an automobile safely for 12 to 24 hours after the time of sedation, they must have a person of driving age accompany them to the MRI facility. If patients appear at the facility without having arranged for a driver or taxi to take them home, they should be rescheduled or allowed to have the examination performed without sedation. It has been suggested that patients who are being sedated be asked to sign a statement indicating that they will not drive an automobile after discharge from the MRI facility. However, this may be of dubious legal value. A judge or jury could later discount the validity of such statements, determining that those made or signed prior to receiving sedating medication were coercive, while those made or signed after receiving sedating medication were invalid because the patient was not sufficiently awake.

Interventional Procedures

Although many practices routinely sedate patients for diagnostic aortofemoral arteriography, the small risk of cardiorespiratory compromise may not be justified in view of the low level of discomfort associated with these procedures.[4] Local anesthesia at the site of catheter insertion is generally sufficient. Conversely, there is a need for sedation and analgesia in patients undergoing therapeutic vascular procedures (e.g., placement of a vena cava filter, TIPS [transjugular intrahepatic portosystem shunt], thrombolysis), which not only are more painful and take longer to perform than routine diagnostic procedures, but also involve catheter exchange and percutaneous dilatation. Similarly, patients for percutaneous catheter biliary or abscess drainage also require sedation and analgesia because of the pain caused by the multiple dilatations through the abdominal or back musculature needed for placement of the large catheters required.[5]

Endnotes

1 Berlin L. Sedation and analgesia in MR imaging. *AJR* 2001;177:293–296.
2 Feinstein KA. Pediatric sedation. In: *Risk Management: Test and Syllabus*. Reston, VA: American College of Radiology, 1999:51–56.
3 Berlin L. Sedation and analgesia in MR imaging. *AJR* 2001;177:293–296.
4 Kennedy PT, Kelly IMG, Loan WC, Boyd CS. Conscious sedation and analgesia for routine aortofemoral arteriography: a prospective evaluation. *Radiology* 2000;216:660–664.
5 Mueller PR, Wittenberg KH, Kaufman JA, Lee MJ. Patterns of anesthesia and nursing care for interventional radiology procedures: a national survey of physician practices and preferences. *Radiology* 1997;202:339–343.

28
Medical Devices

The marketing of medical devices within the United States is governed by the Food, Drug, and Cosmetic Act (FDCA), as modified by the Medical Device Amendments of 1976. It defines a medical device as any health care product that does not achieve its principal, intended purposes by chemical action in or on the body or being metabolized (i.e., not a drug). Administering the act falls under the purview of the Food and Drug Administration (FDA), which bears the responsibility of ensuring that medical devices are both safe and effective for their intended use. In addition to the marketing of medical devices, the FDA also approves and inspects manufacturing of the product, packages inserts, and therapeutic claims of efficacy.[1]

The FDA regulatory system divides medical devices into two groups—those marketed before 1976 ("pre-amendment devices") and those marketed after that date. Pre-1976 devices are divided into three classes related to the potential risk they pose to patients. Class I refers to relatively simple items with minimal if any risk, such as tongue depressors and crutches. They require merely the "general controls" that apply to all medical devices, such as proper registration, record keeping, and labeling. Class I devices must be "safe and effective" for their approved use, but FDA approval is given for general categories of products as a group rather than for those specifically made by an individual manufacturer. Class II devices pose a greater risk of harm and thus are subject to "special controls," such as performance standards, market surveillance, patient registries, guidelines, recommendations, and other appropriate actions. Although the regulations are stricter, they still are applied only to general categories of products. Examples of class II devices are catheters, tampons, cardiac monitors, and oxygen masks. Class III medical devices, which include implanted and life-supporting or life-sustaining devices (heart valves, stents, angioplasty catheters, coils for embolization) are subject to premarket approval for their safety and efficacy, unless the FDA determines that such approval is unnecessary.[2,3]

The classification of a medical device marketed after passage of the 1976 amendments depends on whether it is considered to be "substantially equivalent" (or an "evolutionary change") to one that existed prior to 1976 or deemed to be a genuinely new product. Substantially equivalent devices are placed in the same regulatory class as the pre-amendment device to which they are comparable. Somewhat surprisingly, a high-risk class III medical device considered as "substantially equivalent" to one marketed before 1976 is "grandfathered" and requires only that the manufacturer comply with FDA general controls; in such cases, the agency does not make any explicit safety or efficacy determination prior to marketing. Conversely, all genuinely new medical devices developed after 1976 are automatically classified as class III and subjected to the formal premarket approval process requiring that the manufacturer conduct clinical trials to give a "reasonable assurance" that the device is "safe and effective" for its intended use, "weighing any probable benefit to health from the device against any probable risk of illness or injury from such use." The extensive regulations associated with clinical trials include limited distribution to clinical investigators; comprehensive, federally mandated informed consent requirements; and oversight by an institutional review board (IRD) at each participating institution. An exception may be made for emergency "compassionate" use, when there is a life-threatening condition that needs immediate treatment; no generally acceptable alternative treatment available; and insufficient time to go through the usual FDA procedures to gain approval for such use.[4]

Off-Label Use

Use of an FDA-approved product for a clinical indication other than those specified in the package insert, commonly known as "off-label" use, raises the malpractice issue of whether such conduct is *negligence per se*—violation of a federal regulation that automatically implies that the physician has fallen below the standard of care. However, courts (and amendments to the FDCA) have consistently ruled that, despite tight FDA regulation of the *marketing* of medical products, once they have been approved for *some* use a practitioner may prescribe the drug or employ the device for an off-label use—the so-called "practice of medicine" exception. Indeed, valid new uses for marketed products are often first discovered by innovative approaches taken by health professionals, which later are confirmed by well-confirmed clinical trials. Before the product's label may be revised to include new indications, the substantiating data must be submitted to the

FDA for review and approval. This process takes time and may never occur, for the manufacturer may be unwilling to spend the large amount of money necessary for full clinical trials. Therefore, accepted medical practice often includes unlabeled uses that are not reflected in the product's current labeling.[5,6]

Off-label use is a common medical practice, especially among interventional radiologists. For example, some may employ a stent with FDA approval for arterial use in the venous system. However, there are some major caveats that should be observed. "Radiologists should use medical devices off-label only for indications that are widely recognized in their specialty. Such off-label indications are commonly described in scientific journals or discussed at professional meetings." The availability of authoritative sources permits the radiologist who uses the product off-label to convincingly argue that such use is within the standard of care, thus refuting the common claim made by a plaintiff's attorney that medical devices lacking FDA approval for a specific cause are experimental.[7]

Use of a medical device for which there is little or no support in general clinical practice and the radiology literature should be undertaken only with great caution. Although such use is not necessarily a violation of applicable FDA regulations, it may expose the radiologist to the charge that the use is experimental or even contraindicated. If the radiologist nevertheless believes that the off-label use is justified because no other option exists, the circumstances supporting the decision should be documented in detail in the patient's chart and the procedure report.[8]

Extensive off-label use of a product that is not generally acknowledged in the radiology community can be fraught with hazard and should be discouraged. A radiologist who is actively promoting this off-label use may be accused of violating FDA regulations that prohibit the marketing of products for nonapproved indications. If there has been actual modification of the medical device, the radiologist could have an increased chance of being dragged into a malpractice lawsuit based on *product liability*. According to this theory, the manufacturer of an "unreasonably dangerous" product is subject to *strict liability*—the plaintiff does not need to show negligence but only that the product was "defective" and that its use resulted in actual damages. A manufacturer subjected to a lawsuit stemming from off-label use of its product could attempt to implicate and bring into the action the physician who actually used the product (even though the plaintiff did not wish to pursue litigation against the physician), claiming that the manufacturer did not market the device for the off-label indication and certainly did not sanction any modification to it. Off-label use whose primary intent is to gather data for gaining FDA approval for the indication may increase the risk of malpractice liability from a plaintiff charging that such conduct required the obtaining of an investigational device exemption from the FDA and adherence to the rigid regulatory requirements covered by such an exemption.[9]

Although practitioners can lawfully use medical devices in an off-label manner, manufacturers of such devices are severely restricted as to what information they may provide physicians about such off-label use. Actively marketing such use or describing the nonsanctioned indication on the package insert is forbidden. Although this policy is designed to ensure that the manufacturer actively seeks formal FDA approval for all clinical indications, it often results in informational material supplied by the manufacturer failing to include all medically accepted uses of the product.[10]

Informed Consent for Off-Label Use

Courts have consistently held that FDA-regulatory status is not a "material risk inherently involved in a proposed therapy which a physician should disclose to a patient" in the process of obtaining informed consent.[11] This is based on a series of cases involving the off-label placement of pedicle screws that had received approval for use elsewhere in the skeleton.[12,13] The underlying purpose of the device—the placement of metallic screws to secure bone—was the same; only the site of use differed.

Nevertheless, radiologists should inform their patients of the non-FDA-approved use of a medical device, especially if they practice in states that follow the "reasonable patient" (minority) rule of informed consent (see page 141), or in "reasonable physician" states if most local radiologists inform their patients of the regulatory status of medical devices used. Radiologists contemplating unusual off-label use of FDA-approved products, or employing products that lack any FDA approval for human use, should definitely provide information to the patient about the regulatory status of the device since courts could well consider them experimental. When using experimental devices distributed under an Investigational Device Exemption, it is mandatory to adhere to the extensive FDA regulations that require an elaborate informed consent process, lest one be in violation of federal law.[14]

Reprocessing and Reuse of Single-Use Devices[15]

Single-use medical devices (e.g., catheters and guidewires commonly used in radiology) "are expensive to purchase and store, typically requiring larger inventories than multiple-use devices. In addition, disposal of increased volumes of medical waste is more costly." As budgetary pressures due to financial restraints have become more onerous, the reprocessing and reuse of single-use medical devices has become commonplace in modern radiology practice. This theoretically poses the threat of an increased risk of patient injury. "Faulty resterilization may lead to the transmission of infectious disease between patients, whereas the reprocessing process itself may alter a device's mechanical properties and thus risk product failure." Catheter or guidewire tips may break off within the patient, leading to catastrophic iatrogenic embolisms. Nevertheless, although some anecdotal reports of patient injuries resulting from reprocessed single-use devices have received extensive coverage in the media, there have been relatively few documented cases of this complication.

Traditionally, the FDA placed responsibility for the safety and effectiveness of reprocessed products on those performing the reprocessing. Because the agency selectively enforced its manufacturing regulations only on third-party reprocessors, hospitals that reprocessed devices in their own facilities were left essentially unregulated. As public concern regarding iatrogenic medical injuries grew in the late 1990s, the FDA issued a revised policy, under which "all reprocessors of single-use devices became subject to the same marketing and manufacturing regulations that applied to original equipment manufacturers."

"Although there is at present no federal or state law or regulation that specifically prohibits the reprocessing and reuse of single-use devices, nonetheless, physicians and medical institutions that indulge in such practices may find themselves subjected to malpractice litigation and liability for any injury sustained by the patient." Although most courts have ruled that physicians do not have to inform a patient that a medical device is being used for a non-FDA-approved indication, reasoning that regulatory status is not relevant to patient risk, the judicial conclusion may be the exact opposite "if an off-label use could be seen as increasing patient risk, such as may be the case with reprocessing and reusing a product labeled for single-use only." Therefore, it may be reasonable for a radiologist to advise the patient in advance that the upcoming procedure will involve the use of a reprocessed product. Radiologists who choose to reuse single-use medical devices must be certain that the reprocessing, whether done by the health care facility or delegated to a third-party reprocessor, is performed in compliance with applicable FDA regulations. Most importantly, "radiologists using a reprocessed device should inspect the device carefully before using it to be reasonably comfortable with the fact that it is intact and undamaged. If a radiologist suspects that a specific reprocessed device is unsafe, the device should not be used."

Endnotes

1 Hoffman FA, Rheinstein PH. Health professionals and the regulated industry: the laws and regulations enforced by the U.S. Food and Drug Administration. In: Sanbar SS, Gibofsky A, Firestone MH, et al (eds). *Legal Medicine, 5th ed*. St. Louis, Mosby, 2001, pgs 578–579.

2 Ibid.

3 Smith JJ. Biliary interventional procedures and use of investigational devices. In: *Risk Management: Test and Syllabus*. Reston, American College of Radiology 1999:95–107.

4 Ibid.

5 Smith JJ, Berlin L. Off-label use of interventional medical devices. *AJR* 1999;173:539–542.

6 Hoffman FA, Rheinstein PH. Health professionals and the regulated industry: the laws and regulations enforced by the U.S. Food and Drug Administration. In: Sanbar SS, Gibofsky A, Firestone MH, et al (eds). *Legal Medicine, 5th ed*. St. Louis, Mosby, 2001, pg 582.

7 Smith JJ, Berlin L. Off-label use of interventional medical devices. *AJR* 1999;173:539–542.

8 Ibid.

9 Ibid.

10 Smith JJ. Biliary interventional procedures and use of investigational devices. In: *Risk Management: Test and Syllabus*. Reston, American College of Radiology 1999:95–188.

11 *Klein et al v Biscup et al*, A3d 855 (Ohio 1996).

12 *Corrigan v Methodist Hospital et al*, WL 686626 (PA 1994).

13 *In re Orthopedic bone screw products liability litigation*, WL 107556 (PA 1996).

14 Smith JJ, Berlin L. Informed consent when using medical devices for indications non approved by the Food and Drug Administration. *AJR* 1999;173:879–882.

15 Smith JJ, Berlin L. Reusing catheters and other medical devices. *AJR* 2001;177:773–776.

29
The Pregnant Patient

Malpractice lawsuits charging that an abortion or fetal anomaly was caused by exposure to diagnostic radiation are infrequent. Nevertheless, radiologists should make every effort to decrease the likelihood of exposing an unknowingly pregnant woman to radiation in order to prevent clinical danger to the fetus and any potential legal liability.[1]

Effect of Radiation Exposure on the Fetus

The relationship between in utero radiation and the development of congenital anomalies is difficult to evaluate because abnormalities can be detected in 5% to 10% of all children who have had no exposure to radiation.[2] It is known that a fetus of between 2 and 15 weeks' gestational age is most sensitive to adverse effects from radiation, especially microcephaly (at times combined with mental retardation), other central nervous system defects, and growth retardation. Radiation-induced abnormalities in fetuses exposed to radiation before 2 weeks' or after 15 weeks' gestation are highly unlikely.[3] "The radiation dose below which no harmful effects on the fetus occur even during the most sensitive developmental phase is not known, but has been estimated to be in the range of 5-15 rad (0.05-0.15 Gy)."[4]

According to the American College of Radiology, "The interruption of pregnancy is rarely justified because of radiation risk to the embryo or fetus from a radiologic examination."[5] One classic text states that there is no indication for a therapeutic abortion if a fetus outside the sensitive time of 2 to 15 weeks' gestation is exposed to a radiation dose of 5 rad or less (and even possibly as high as 15 rad).[6] Another authority suggests that termination of the pregnancy should be considered if a fetus of 10 days' to 26 weeks' gestational age has received a radiation dose of 10 rad.[7] Even if the radiation exposure exceeds these levels, a recommendation to terminate pregnancy should be based on additional factors, such as "the hazard of pregnancy to the expectant mother, the ethnic and religious background of the family and their attitudes toward possibly bearing a child with a congenital deformity, state law regarding abortion, genetic factors, age of the mother, and any associated clinical diseases or conditions."[8]

Determining Whether a Woman Is Pregnant

Surprisingly, "no governmental regulation or formal professional standard absolutely requires that radiologists determine in advance of a radiologic procedure whether a woman of child-bearing age is pregnant." Nevertheless, radiologists should make reasonable efforts to secure this information. Radiology requisition forms to be filled out by referring physicians should include a section dealing with the possibility of pregnancy. Signs should be posted in plain view throughout the waiting and examining areas of the radiology department stating something like, "If you are pregnant or think you might be pregnant, please notify a technologist or physician." Before performing any radiologic examination, technologists should routinely ask women patients whether they are or could be pregnant.[9]

Examining the Pregnant Patient

Radiologic facilities should have a protocol for the management of patients who are pregnant, or indicate that they might be pregnant, to decide prospectively whether they should undergo a radiologic examination. To make this determination, it is necessary to know the gestational age of the fetus and the radiation dose to be received. Fetal age can be determined by the referring physician; an estimation of the radiation dosage related to the specific procedure is the responsibility of the radiologist or medical physicist, who can easily obtain this information from published sources. A radiologist or radiation physicist should be available to discuss with the patient and referring physician the risks of radiation exposure, any danger related to postponing or canceling the radiologic examination, and alternative diagnostic imaging modalities that could be employed. If the decision is made to perform the study, the examination should be modified to reduce the amount of radiation exposure by decreasing the number of radiographic views and shortening any fluoroscopy time.[10]

Radionuclide Imaging

The administration of radioactive iodine to a pregnant woman is known to have harmful effects on the thyroid gland of the fetus. The fetal thyroid gland begins to function at 8 to 14 weeks' gestational age,[11,12] and its capacity to concentrate and store iodine and thyroid hormones increases progressively until birth.[13] The concentration of radioactive iodine in the thyroid gland of the fetus has been reported to be 10 to 50 times that of its mother's.[14,15] Because of the danger of causing severe hypothyroidism at birth, the American College of Radiology explicitly states that iodine-131 is contraindicated during pregnancy.[16] If a radio-nuclide study is absolutely necessary for the clinical welfare of the mother, the agent of choice is iodine-123, which generates only 1% of the radiation exposure.[17]

As with other radiologic studies, radiologists in the nuclear medicine department should actively attempt to determine whether women of childbearing age are pregnant, utilizing the requisition form, posted signs, and direct questioning by the technologist. Because radionuclide studies with iodine-131 (and even iodine-123) entail a high, focused dose to the fetal thyroid gland, it may be wise to have the patient complete and sign a questionnaire that includes a question concerning the possibility of her being pregnant. Such documentation can prevent a subsequent debate as to whether the technologist actually asked the patient about her possible pregnant status. If asked orally whether she could be pregnant, the patient's specific response and the name of the questioner should be documented in writing.[18] Because of the much higher amount of radiation involved, one author[19] has suggested that "it is prudent policy to require a negative pregnancy test before administering therapeutic doses of iodine-131," though this is infrequently done in practice.

The precise likelihood of hypothyroidism actually developing in infants whose mothers inadvertently received iodine-131 for a diagnostic study during pregnancy is unknown. Nevertheless, in a malpractice lawsuit the plaintiff's attorney may well be able to successfully convince a lay judge or jury that a direct cause-and-effect relationship exists between the development of neonatal hypothyroidism and a maternal radionuclide examination during pregnancy.[20]

Endnotes

1 Berlin L. Radiation exposure and the pregnant patient. *AJR* 1996;167:1377–1379.
2 Hall EJ. *Radiobiology for the Radiologist*, 4th ed. Philadelphia: Lippincott, 1994:363–378,419–452.

3 Wagner LK, Lester RG, Saldana LR. *Exposure of the Pregnant Patient to Diagnostic Radiations: A Guide to Medical Management*. Philadelphia: Lippincott, 1985.

4 Berlin L. Radiation exposure and the pregnant patient. *AJR* 1996;167:1377–1379.

5 *ACR Standard for Abdominal Radiologic Examination of Women of Child-Bearing Age and Potential*. Reston, VA: American College of Radiology, 1988.

6 Wagner LK, Lester RG, Saldana LR. *Exposure of the Pregnant Patient to Diagnostic Radiations: A Guide to Medical Management*. Philadelphia: Lippincott, 1985.

7 Hall EJ. *Radiobiology for the Radiologist*, 4th ed. Philadelphia: Lippincott, 1994:363–378, 419–452.

8 Berlin L. Radiation exposure and the pregnant patient. *AJR* 1996;167:1377-1379.

9 Ibid.

10 Ibid.

11 Wagner LK, Lester RG, Saldana LR. *Exposure of the Pregnant Patient to Diagnostic Radiations: A Guide to Medical Management*. Philadelphia: Lippincott, 1985:17–19, 55–57.

12 Hamill GC, Jarman JA, Wynne MD. Fetal effects of radioactive iodine therapy in a pregnant woman with thyroid cancer. *Am J Obstet Gynecol* 1961;81:1018–1023.

13 Harbert JC. Radioiodine therapy of differentiated thyroid carcinoma. In: Harbert JC, Eckelman WC, Neuman RD, eds. *Nuclear Medicine: Diagnosis and Therapy*. New York: Thieme, 1996:1006–1008.

14 Green HG, Gareis FJ, Shepard TH, Kelley VC. Cretinism associated with maternal sodium I-131 therapy during pregnancy. *Am J Dis Child* 1971;122:247–249.

15 Russell KP, Rose H, Starr P. The effects of radioactive iodine on maternal and fetal thyroid function during pregnancy. *Surg Gynecol Obstet* 1957;104:560–564.

16 American College of Radiology. *Radiation Risk: A Primer*. Reston, VA: American College of Radiology 1996:5–10.

17 Berlin L. Iodine-131 and the pregnant patient. *AJR* 2001;176:869–871.

18 Ibid.

19 Harbert JC. Radioiodine therapy of hyperthyroidism. In: Harbert JC, Eckelman WC, Neuman RD, eds. *Nuclear Medicine: Diagnosis and Therapy*. New York: Thieme, 1996:951–965.

20 Berlin L. Iodine-131 and the pregnant patient. *AJR* 2001;176:869–871.

30
Computed Tomography Screening Studies

Computed tomography, especially of the lung for cancer, the heart for coronary artery disease, and the abdomen for any abnormality (degenerative, metabolic, vascular, or neoplastic), has become a hot commodity among the more entrepreneurial members of the radiology community. Unlike conventional radiology practice, in which patients are referred by other physicians, CT screening is usually performed on self-referred patients in response to radio or newspapers advertisements that tout these expensive examinations, which are not covered by medical insurance and usually require an up-front payment by cash or credit card.[1] The text and headlines of these advertisements explicitly or implicitly imply that the accuracy of screening CT is almost 100% and that the early detection of lung cancer or coronary artery disease will ensure a cure. However, as of yet "there is still no proof that CT screening is of any real value or benefit to the patient … [and this technique] is being promoted and performed with little or no scientific evidence to justify or validate such screening."[2] Consequently, patients who reasonably expect that CT screening will always detect and permit cure of disease at its earliest stage may well decide to file a malpractice lawsuit if these expectations are not met.[3]

General Criteria for Effective Screening[4]

"To justify the cost of screening, the target disease should have serious consequences, such as high morbidity or mortality, and a high prevalence of a detectable pre-clinical phase. The screening test itself should have a high sensitivity for detecting disease before the critical point (i.e., the point when it is widespread or metastasizes) [and] a high specificity (i.e., low frequency of detecting pseudo-disease)." Pseudo-disease represents a preclinical condition that would not have produced any symptoms before the person died from some other cause.[5] A negative test should allow patients to feel reasonable comfortable that they are free of disease. Conversely, a screening test must have a low rate of false positives so that healthy persons are not subjected to unwarranted anxiety or to the additional cost and potential morbidity of unnecessary tests or procedures. As a *New York Times* editorial observed,[6] "A key issue [in screening] is whether the tests are finding a lot of tumors that would never become dangerous but cannot be distinguished from tumors that could become deadly, thereby causing many patients to undergo the risk of surgery, radiation or chemotherapy for no good reason." Screening tests must be readily available, reasonably priced, and associated with low morbidity. It is critical to remember that the mere detection of disease is not sufficient for screening; there must be an effective treatment that is not too risky or toxic.

Radiation Risk[7]

The multidetector scanners used in screening CT studies result in patients receiving radiation doses that are about 30% to 50% higher than those with older, single-detector equipment. Reasons for this increase in radiation dosage include scan overlap, positioning of the x-ray tube closer to the patient, and the greater scattered radiation that results with the use of wider x-ray beams. Although it is highly controversial whether the radiation exposure from CT screening will increase the incidence of cancer in the general population, some radiologists have expressed concern and have suggested ways of decreasing radiation exposure, such as by lowering the milliampere-seconds and voltage and increasing the pitch. One article goes so far as to recommended that, before undergoing screening CT, patients should receive information about potential cancer and other radiation risks associated with the procedure. Although there is no scientific proof of specific radiation-induced complications of CT screening, it is reasonable to expect that some enterprising attorney will soon file a medical malpractice action on behalf of a plaintiff alleging that he or she developed a malignancy consequent to the screening CT examination. Although this would probably be dismissed by the court in view of the long latency time for radiation-induced tumors, a much more serious charge would be a woman who claims that she gave birth to a baby with congenital anomalies related to her having undergone a screening CT study at a time when she did not realize that she was pregnant.

CT Screening for Lung Cancer

Although intuitively it makes sense that earlier detection of lung cancer will result in decreased mortality, this assumption has not been proven.[8] One study[9] found no relationship between tumors ≤3 cm in diameter and survival; patients with 3-cm masses had survival rates identical to those with 1-cm nodules. In a related study,[10] there was no correlation between the stage at presentation and the size of the tumor. As one radiologist wrote about CT screening for lung cancer in a major newspaper, "Our ability to discover early-stage tumors or other suspicious lesions is of less-clear value. In some instances, we are clearly discovering slow-growing cancers that will never actually kill the patient, or rapidly growing cancers that have already spread and are thus not early at all."[11]

Computed tomography screening can result in "overdiagnosis"—the detection of small well-differentiated adenocarcinomas that are associated with longer survival.[12] Autopsy studies have shown that one sixth of lung cancers were neither clinically recognized nor the cause of the patient's death.[13] "If CT screening leads to an overdiagnosis of lung cancer, one would expect increases in stage I disease, an increase in resectability, an increase in 5-year survival, and an increase in the total number of cancers but no change in the number of advanced cancers and no decrease in lung cancer deaths." This is precisely what was found in the Mayo Lung Project from the 1970s for screening with chest radiography. Computed tomography is more sensitive than chest radiography for the detection of early lung cancer, but it is unclear whether it will be any more effective as a screening technique. Computed tomography screening may merely be detecting even more lesions of no clinical significance that necessitate expensive follow-up, needless patient worry, or even unnecessary surgery.[14]

What is the expected "miss rate" of carcinomas on chest CT? In a controlled study, experienced thoracic radiologists aware that each case contained a missed cancer still were unable to detect it more than half the time.[15] Similarly, another article reported that half the lung cancers detected on CT were present (but missed) on a previous CT screening examination.[16] These failures to detect lung carcinoma have been attributed to lack of conspicuity and technical factors, such as partial volume averaging and misregistration,[17] and to the problem of prominent blood vessels and that large amount of data that can lead to "information overload."[18] Regardless of the underlying cause, the message is clear: it is inevitable than some small carcinomas will not be identified on screening chest CT and thus may serve as the subject for subsequent litigation by patients who were convinced by high-profile advertising that every malignant chest lesion would be detected by this technique.[19] One suggested approach to decrease the number of false negatives is the use of some method of computerized nodule detection to serve as a "second reader." This could help radiologists "focus their attention on regions that might contain lung cancer" as well as "direct radiologists to suspicious lesions that would merit immediate examination with targeted full-dose thin-section CT after having been detected during an initial low-dose [screening] CT scan."[20]

Patients may suffer several potential harmful effects from screening CT for lung cancer.[21] These include "complications from biopsies required for false-positive findings; morbidity and mortality of surgery performed for questionably malignant or minimally malignant lesions; and excessive radiation exposure due to the multiple high-resolution CT follow-up examinations of patients in whom tiny non-calcified nodules are found."[22]

Serious ethical questions, primarily involving informed consent, have been raised about advertising the alleged benefits of CT screening to the general public in the United States. The claim that lung cancer can be found at its earliest stage would reasonably lead to the assumption that CT screening can save a person's life—a claim that a layperson would presume was based on extensive scientific studies. However, the advertisement is based not on evidence-based medicine but on entrepreneurial promotion by radiologists and other physicians who stand to make a financial windfall from the procedure. As Swensen wrote, "The bottom line is that we are unequivocally required as scientists and health professionals to thoroughly study this new `beast' before jumping into what might be a quagmire. A randomized, controlled trial is the best way to address the controversy and probably the only way that third-party payers will ever agree to pay for this screening—if a trial shows positive results."[23]

CT Screening for Coronary Artery Disease

The rationale for CT screening of the heart is based on research and autopsy studies that have demonstrated a relationship between the presence of occlusive coronary artery disease and coronary artery calcification.[24] The current concept is that the quantity of calcified plaque indicates the presence and amount of soft, relatively unstable plaque that is most likely to rupture and cause myocardial infarction.[25] The absence of coronary artery calcification means that the patient has a low risk of future serious cardiac events (negative predictive value estimated at 90% to 95%).[26] Therefore, some authorities have suggested CT examination of the heart to be of particular value in assessing otherwise healthy patients who complain of acute chest pain. One study of patients admitted to hospital emergency rooms with chest pain reported a negligible risk of immediate myocardial infarction in those who had negative findings on heart CT. Moreover, the future annual rate of sustaining a serious cardiac event was substantially below 1%.[27] However, although patients with negative heart CT scans have a decreased incidence of cardiac events, when they do occur they are apt to be catastrophic.[28]

Computed tomography screening of the heart can accurately detect the presence of calcium, which is a marker of coronary artery occlusive disease. Patients without detectable calcium have a low probability of undergoing future cardiac events. However, "as many as 10% of screened patients with no demonstrable calcium may suffer a perhaps severe and possibly fatal myocardial infarction."[29] Some patients (or their estates) in this category will undoubtedly file malpractice suits claiming erroneous interpretation of the screening CT study, arguing that the natural history of coronary artery disease indicates that these vessels must have been diseased at the time of the examination but not properly imaged due to negligence on the part of the radiologist.

CT Screening for Abdominal Pathology[30]

Baker has raised numerous issues concerning the practice of screening studies for detecting abdominal pathology in asymptomatic individuals. On the nonenhanced studies used for screening, the diagnostic value of CT is inherently limited because of a lack of opacification of both the parenchyma and adjacent vascular structures. Moreover, in some conditions CT is no more effective than sonography, which is less expensive and does not use ionizing radiation.

For carcinomas of the prostate and cervix/uterus, nonimaging studies (serum prostate-specific antigen (PSA) levels and rectal palpation; Pap smear) are the major screening tests. Carcinomas of the stomach, pancreas, and gallbladder are extremely difficult to detect at an early stage and are not typically present in asymptomatic individuals. Abdominal node enlargement is rarely the initial presentation of non-Hodgkin's lymphomas; hepatomas rarely occur in persons without known risk factors and usually can only be detected on contrast-enhanced scans. Adrenal carcinomas are slow-growing and may be detected at an early stage, but "in the United States, fewer than 500 individuals die from this malignancy annually" and "by consensus, adrenal tumors smaller than 3 cm are usually left untreated." Renal carcinoma typically causes hematuria, palpable flank mass, or fever. "Unless a [renal] carcinoma is large enough to protrude well beyond the renal contours (which makes it also more likely to have already metastasized), the carcinoma is apt to be missed if no contrast material is used."

Although it is true that nonenhanced screening CT could reveal calcification in the aorta and iliac arteries, this is not an unequivocal indication of similar involvement of the arteries supplying the heart and brain. Furthermore, "it is not necessarily true that the absence of calcification in the abdominal arteries can serve as indicator of vascular health elsewhere in the body." Computed tomography even without contrast can detect abdominal aneurysms, but these are highly unlikely in patients under than age 60 who have no known risk factors (hypertension, arteriosclerosis, history of smoking); even when they occur, sonography would be equally effective for revealing an abdominal aneurysm.

Use of Contrast Material in Screening CT Studies[31]

According to the American College of Radiology (ACR) Standard for Performing and Interpreting Diagnostic Computed Tomography (CT),[32] "The physician shall have the responsibility for reviewing all indications for the examination, specifying the use, dosage, and rate of administration of contrast agents." This standard was developed for symptomatic patients referred to radiologists by nonradiologist physicians who have examined the patient. With reference to whole-body screening CT, there is still no consensus as to whether contrast material is indicated. Currently, most radiologists do not administer contrast material, primarily due to the fear of potential complications. However, some advocate including the administration of contrast material as part of their standard protocol for CT screening.[33] Either choice could potentially result in liability. As Berlin has observed, "If contrast material is not used and a small carcinoma of an abdominal or pelvic organ is missed, a plaintiff's attorney may well be able to find a well-credentialed radiology expert who will testify that the standard of care requires the use of contrast media in CT screening." Conversely, if contrast material is used and results in death or a serious nonfatal complication, it would be relatively easy to find an equally well-credentialed radiologist to state at trial that "the standard of care requires that radiologists not administer contrast media when performing CT screening."

Medical-Legal Implications[34]

Berlin has extensively explored the legal ramifications of CT screening procedures. He observes that "radiologists who decide to advertise CT lung or heart screening, or who prepare written literature for patients undergoing such screening, should be extremely cautious about the content of such material. Radiologists should be wary of making misrepresentations that cannot be proven, such as that the test will detect all early abnormalities or that the detection of a disease at an early stage will assure a cure of that disease." Despite the fact that advertisements are designed to solicit patients into undergoing CT screening by emphasizing only the potential benefits of the studies, radiologists should realize that they also "have an obligation to present information or to discuss with patients the benefits, risks, and non-monetary as well as monetary costs of the tests in question," including "any potential negative consequences that may result from the testing." Failure to do this could leave radiologists exposed to charges of misrepresentation and lack of informed consent.

Another serious potential problem is that radiologists who perform CT screening on self-referred patients must realize that "they are establishing a physician-patient relationship … and thereby may have imposed upon themselves the duty not only to communicate results of the examination directly to patients, but also to be responsible for follow-up care of the patient, particularly if the screening yields positive findings." Failure to accomplish these tasks may result in legal liability for patient abandonment.

Endnotes

1 Berlin L. Liability of performing CT screening for coronary artery disease and lung cancer. *AJR* 2002;179:837–842.
2 Rogers LF. Whole-body CT screening: edging toward commerce. *AJR* 2002;179:823.
3 Berlin L. Liability of performing CT screening for coronary artery disease and lung cancer. *AJR* 2002;179:837–842.
4 Siegel MJ. CT screening for cancer. *RadioGraphics* 2002;22:1521–1523.
5 Black WC, Welch HG. Screening for disease. *AJR* 1997;186:3–11.
6 Cancer screening and the individual (editorial). *New York Times*, April 14, 2002:12.
7 Berlin B. Potential legal ramifications of whole-body CT screening: taking a peek into Pandora's box. *AJR* 2003;180:317–322.
8 Swensen SJ. CT screening for lung cancer. *AJR* 2002;179:833–836.
9 Patz EF JR, Rossi S, Harpole DH, et al. Correlation of tumor size and survival in patients with stage 1A non-small cell lung cancer. *Chest* 2000;117:1568–1571.
10 Heyneman LE, Herndon E, Goodman PC, Patz EF Jr. Stage distribution in patients with a small (< or = 3 cm) primary nonsmall cell lung carcinoma: implication for lung carcinoma screening. *Cancer* 2001;92:3051–3055.
11 Lerner BH. Screening for cancer: a downside. *New York Times*, March 5, 2002:D6.
12 Swensen SJ. CT screening for lung cancer. *AJR* 2002;179:833–836.

13 Chan CK, Wells CK, McFarlane MJ, Feinstein AR. More lung cancer but better survival: implications of secular trends in "necropsy surprise" rates. *Chest* 1989;96:291–296.

14 Swensen SJ. CT screening for lung cancer. *AJR* 2002;179:833–836.

15 White CS, Romney BM, Mason AC, et al. Primary carcinoma of the lung overlooked at CT: analysis of findings in 14 patients. *Radiology* 1996; 199:109–115.

16 Kakinuma R, Ohmatsu H, Kaneko M, et al. Detection failure in spiral CT screening for lung cancer: analysis of CT findings. *Radiology* 1999;212: 61–66.

17 White CS, Romney BM, Mason AC, et al. Primary carcinoma of the lung overlooked at CT: analysis of findings in 14 patients. *Radiology* 1996; 199:109–115.

18 Armato SG III, Li F, Giger ML, et al. Lung cancer: performance of automated lung nodule detection applied to cancers missed in a CT screening program. *Radiology* 2002;225:685–692.

19 Berlin L. Liability of performing CT screening for coronary artery disease and lung cancer. *AJR* 2002;179:837–842.

20 Armato SG III, Li F, Giger ML, et al. Lung cancer: performance of automated lung nodule detection applied to cancers missed in a CT screening program. *Radiology* 2002;225:685–692.

21 Frame PS. Routine screening for lung cancer? Maybe someday but not yet. *JAMA* 2000;284:1980–1983.

22 Berlin L. Liability of performing CT screening for coronary artery disease and lung cancer. *AJR* 2002;179:837–842.

23 Swensen SJ. CT screening for lung cancer. *AJR* 2002;179:833–836.

24 Breen JF, Sheedy PF, Schwartz RS, et al. Coronary artery calcification detected with ultrafast CT as an indication of coronary artery disease. *Radiology* 1992;185:435–439.

25 Budoff MJ. Prognostic value of coronary artery calcification. *J Clin Outcomes Manage* 2001;8:42–48.

26 Stanford W, Thompson BH. Imaging of coronary artery calcification. *Radiol Clin North Am* 1999;37:257–272.

27 Georgiou D, Budoff J, Kaufer E, et al. Screening patients with chest pain in the emergency department using electron beam tomography: a follow-up study. *J Am Coll Cardiol* 2001;38:105–110.

28 Berlin L. Liability of performing CT screening for coronary artery disease and lung cancer. *AJR* 2002;179:837–842.

29 Ibid.

30 Baker SR. Abdominal CT screening: inflated promises, serious concerns. *AJR* 2003;180:27–30.

31 Berlin L. Should whole-body CT screening be performed with contrast media? *AJR* 2003;180:323–325.

32 American College of Radiology. Standard for performing and interpret-

ing diagnostic computed tomography (CT). In: *Standards 2001–2002.* Reston, VA: American College of Radiology, 2001:37–40.

33 Fishman EK, Horton KM. Screening strategy joins contrast, noncontrast scans. *Diagn Imaging* 2002;24:45,47.

34 Berlin L. Liability of performing CT screening for coronary artery disease and lung cancer. *AJR* 2002;179:837–842.

Part V
Electronic Imaging

31
Teleradiology

The electronic transmission of radiologic images has raised a host of medical-legal issues, many of which have not yet been addressed in actual lawsuits. However, it is possible to make reasonable predictions of how courts will rule on these issues by making analogies to other situations with well-developed case law.

Establishment of Physician-Patient Relationship

To succeed in a medical malpractice lawsuit, the plaintiff must demonstrate the existence of a physician-patient relationship. In radiology, this was traditionally proven when the radiologist rendered a formal interpretation of a patient's imaging examination, regardless of whether the two had ever actually met. Once the physician-patient relationship is established, the physician owes the patient the duty to exercise reasonable skill and knowledge; any breach of that duty exposes the radiologist to liability for malpractice.

In the context of teleradiology (and other forms of telemedicine), there may be only a computer interaction between a patient and a distant consultant, often with a local physician acting as an intermediary. If radiologists are providing official interpretations of imaging studies, such as on-call radiologists at home interpreting after-hours examinations sent from their facilities, a physician-patient relationship is clearly established. In the case of "nighthawks"—distant radiologists, unrelated to the facility, who interpret examinations after hours—the fact that the emergency medicine physicians or other referring clinicians materially relied on their opinions in diagnosing and treating their patients should be sufficient to establish a physician-patient relationship. However, if the distant radiologist is only acting in the role of a consultant to a locally licensed radiologist, it may be unclear whether a physician-patient relationship exists. Such an informal "curbside" consultation (see page 4) may not be sufficient to establish a physician-patient relationship unless it can be shown that the local radiologist materially relied on the consulting radiologist's opinion in rendering his or her own formal interpretation.

Medical Licensing and Insurance[1,2]

Each state has enacted laws and established medical boards that govern the licensing of physicians practicing within its boundaries. Physicians who practice without valid licenses are subject to civil fines, exclusion from federal Medicare and Medicaid programs, and even criminal penalties. Most states permit unlicensed out-of-state physicians to enter their state for "occasional" consultations, provided that these consultants confer with a local physician who is appropriately licensed in the state. However, state laws vary as to how frequently such consultations can occur without the out-of-state physician being required to secure a local license. Several states have "border states exceptions," which exempt licensed physicians in immediately neighboring states from the state's licensure requirements.

The rise of telemedicine and its potential to create competition between in-state licensed physicians and out-of-state unlicensed physicians has changed the regulatory landscape. No longer is it necessary for the out-of-state physician to physically enter the local state; distant physicians can remotely render patient care locally without ever leaving the computer monitor in their homes. In response to the demands of local physicians to protect their turf, most states mandate that physicians who practice telemedicine from remote locations must be fully licensed in both the state where the physician resides and the state in which the image originated. This generally is justified by deeming the practice of medicine a "privilege" and requiring local licensure so that the state has the ability to discipline practitioners when "necessary for the public health, welfare and safety,"[3] thus providing for effective quality control and accountability.

Today, licensure requirements for out-of-state teleradiology practitioners fall into three general categories: (a) full licensure is either expressly required by statute or presumed because teleradiology and/or telemedicine is not specifically mentioned in the applicable medical practice act and no exemption applies (by far the majority of states); (b) a "special purpose" license for out-of-state teleradiology practitioners is available; and (c) full licensure is not required, though something short of full licensure may be necessary. Obviously, it is critical for anyone contemplating the practice of teleradiology to be certain of the licensure requirements in any state(s) from which images will be originating.

The time and cost required to obtain and maintain medical licenses in multiple states has succeeded in limiting the spread of teleradiology services. It also has raised the significant issue of whether those physicians practicing teleradiology are covered by their professional insurance carriers. Coverage of out-of-state teleradiology activities should not be assumed. Not all insurance carriers are licensed in every state, and underwriting criteria between jurisdictions may vary. Accordingly, many malpractice policies specifically exclude coverage for out-of-state incidents, unless a rider has been added to specifically provide such coverage. This means that unwary teleradiology practitioners subject to an out-of-state malpractice action may find their professional liability carriers limiting or even completely denying coverage.

Teleradiologists must also abide by the credentialing requirements of the specific health care facilities for which they are providing services. In addition, new stringent privacy laws require that teleradiologists develop security procedures to prevent unauthorized access to the medical information related to their electronic images.

Jurisdiction for Malpractice Suits[4]

If a physician practicing teleradiology is sued for malpractice, where should the case be heard? Traditionally, this has not posed a problem since the appropriate jurisdiction was the state in which the patient was injured and the physician practiced medicine. However, the interstate practice of telemedicine has given plaintiffs the opportunity to "forum shop"—to sue in the state that is most advantageous to their cases with regard to such factors (varying among the states) as the statute of limitations, procedural and evidentiary rules, and the existence of statutory caps on malpractice awards. In most cases, state courts claim jurisdiction in cases involving medical injuries suffered by residents of their states. Some states have enacted legislation that specifically subjects out-of-state telemedicine practitioners to the jurisdiction of that state's court system. This means that teleradiologists may be forced to defend themselves in a distant locality, resulting in substantial travel costs, forcing them to be away from home for a considerable time, and depriving them of any protections (such as limits on the amounts of malpractice awards) that they enjoy in their home states.

Other Medical-Legal Aspects[5,6]

Those involved in teleradiology—both the local health care facility and the remote radiologist—have a duty to maintain the equipment in good working condition and to use it appropriately. The manufacturer or vendor of the teleradiology equipment may be subject to product liability if a malfunction occurs. Professional personnel at the sending or receiving site may be liable if density settings and other computer parameters, such as the speed of transmission and compression of data, are not adjusted appropriately and result in degraded images that are not interpreted properly and lead to patient injury. Telemedicine technologies may suffer intermittent failures, especially those that depend on satellite links. Other still-undetermined issues are whether the electronic information or the hardcopy (or both) constitutes the original medical record that must be retained by the radiologic facility, and the extent of safeguards that must be created to prevent tampering with the original electronic information.

As teleradiology becomes generally adopted in the medical community, failure to obtain a subspecialty consultation or definitive reading of a complex set of images may be viewed as violating the standard of care, when such consultation is readily available using telemedicine technology.

Relationship Between Local and Distant Radiologists

Many radiologists view teleradiologists as posing a direct threat to their livelihood. There are valid fears that managed care plans or independent hospitals will use teleradiology to replace local radiologists with out-of-state radiology groups. Indeed, there are teleradiology companies that offer services in direct competition with local radiologists in both rural and metropolitan areas throughout the United States.[7] Although some have argued that such developments only improve patient care by allowing "the transmission of images in difficult cases to those members of a group best trained to interpret them,"[8] others have maintained that teleradiology should be used only to enhance one's own practice and "not to invade the practice of another radiologist."[9]

Local animosity can adversely affect teleradiologists in subtle ways. The displacement of existing hospital radiologists could lead to antagonism toward the "interlopers" by local radiology personnel and nonradiology medical staff physicians. Conceivably, this resentment could undermine the performance of the teleradiology group and increase its exposure to liability. Moreover, should malpractice litigation be instituted, teleradiologists may find it difficult to present an effective defense. Local juries may be biased against "foreigners" who are perceived as having thrown out those radiologists who had long served their community with distinction. In addition, these displaced local radiologists probably would be extremely willing to testify as expert witnesses for the plaintiff.[10]

Endnotes

1 Berlin L. Teleradiology. *AJR* 1998;170:1417–1422.

2 Smith JJ, Zibners H. Legal issues and formal policies. In: Dreyer KJ, Mehta A, Thrall JH, eds. *PACS: A Guide to the Digital Revolution*. New York, Springer, 2002:351–373.

3 Telemedicine Licensing Act. Illinois Senate Bill 314 (July 11, 1997).

4 Berlin L. Teleradiology. *AJR* 1998;170:1417–1422.

5 Ibid.

6 Kuszler PC. Telemedicine and integrated health care delivery: compounding medical liability. *Am J Law Med Ethics* 1999;25:297–325.

7 Berlin L. Teleradiology. *AJR* 1998;170:1417–1422.

8 Casarella WJ. Benefits of teleradiology. *Radiology* 1996;201:16.

9 Lee CD. Teleradiology. *Radiology* 1996;201:15.

10 Berlin L. Teleradiology. *AJR* 1998;170:1417–1422.

32
E-Mail

As e-mail becomes progressively more popular as a means of communication, radiologists as well as other physicians are likely to be subjected to increased levels of electronic messages from both known patients and unknown others seeking medical advice. Radiologists without direct patient-care responsibility may receive e-mail from patients who discover their names on radiology reports. "Those who list their names on a Web site, those in academic settings, and those who become recognized for certain specific procedures or examinations can well expect to receive e-mail communications relating to their practice from a variety of sources." When deciding how to respond to the "medical questions posed in such messages, radiologists should be mindful that the legal standards applied to everyday medical practice also apply to e-mail consultation."[1]

From the legal point of view, e-mail messages are analogous to telephone conversations, since both are electronic communications in which the parties do not have to be within physical proximity. As with other aspects of malpractice law, an essential issue is whether a radiologist's response to an unsolicited e-mail from an unknown patient, or from another physician regarding an unknown patient, establishes a physician-patient relationship. Case law has clearly indicated that this requires a "consensual relationship in which the patient knowingly seeks the physician's assistance and the physician knowingly accepts the person as a patient.... A doctor who gives an informal opinion at the request of a treating physician does not owe a duty of care to the patient whose case was discussed."[2] Merely engaging in a telephone conversation with a patient is not sufficient to form a physician–patient relationship as long as the physician does not provide any medical advice, "for there is no rule that requires a physician to undertake the treatment of every patient who applies to him."[3] Instead, a physician must indicate, either implicitly or explicitly, a willingness to enter into such a relationship.[4]

Although there is no directly applicable case law, by extension it would seem reasonable to assume that a radiologist is under no obligation to respond to an unsolicited e-mail communication, regardless of its content. However, it is likely that a physician-patient relationship would be created if a radiologist does reply to an unsolicited e-mail and offers medical advice such as a diagnosis or an opinion as to what additional imaging studies may be necessary.[5] Similarly, if a radiologist receives an unsolicited message from another physician regarding a patient unknown to the radiologist and either does not respond or merely sends a courteous reply that does not include specific medical advice, no physician-patient relationship would be established. However, as with "curbside" consultations either in person or by telephone, if the radiologist sends a return e-mail that provides medical advice on which the consulting physician relies in treating the patient, a court may well deem that a requisite physician–patient relationship exists.[6]

Radiologists who respond to medical questions posed in e-mail messages must remember that they will be subject to the same standard of care as in traditional forms of communication. Therefore, as Smith and Berlin have concluded, "a radiologist who relies on a patient's written description of radiologic findings [in an e-mail] and then offers an incorrect diagnosis based only on that description would probably not be acting within the standard of care. Conversely, a radiologist who responds to a similarly vague e-mail query by demanding a firsthand viewing of the radiographic images before rendering an opinion, offering the patient an opportunity for a formal in-person consultation, or referring the patient to a competent licensed radiologist in the patient's community, is unlikely to be found negligent." In general, the basic criterion determining liability should be whether the radiologist rendered an opinion that was reasonable given the amount of information provided.

It is dangerous for radiologists to offer opinions or other medical advice based on the limited information provided in an e-mail, especially if based solely on the patient's description of imaging or clinical findings. This is of special concern since e-mail provides a reproducible written record of the original message and the radiologist's response.[8] Although it would seem to be a matter of common sense that physicians should not go out on a limb providing diagnoses and advice based solely on information supplied in an unsolicited e-mail, published reports have shown that this is not necessarily the case. In one study,[9] 50% of dermatologists responded to an e-mail regarding infection by herpes zoster in a fictitious patient on immunosuppressive therapy. Of these, 59% (30% of those who received the e-mail) explicitly mentioned the correct "diagnosis" in their reply despite the obvious danger of misdiagnosis in the absence of access to a complete patient history and physical examination. Although ignoring an unsolicited e-mail is clearly the safest course of action, those radiologists who feel duty bound to reply should consider a response similar to one suggested by a group of British orthopaedic surgeons:[10]

"I am sorry but I cannot answer unsolicited questions sent from patients or relatives to me either by e-mail or through my Web site. Clinical advice must be obtained from your general practitioner or surgeon. Unsolicited e-mails asking for medical advice, surgical or physician referrals, and sources of medical information will not be answered."

Other Potential Problems with E-Mail

As in the setting of teleradiology, offering medical advice by e-mail to out-of-state patients could be interpreted as practicing medicine without a license in the state where the patient resides, if the radiologist lacks a valid license in that jurisdiction.[11] Although generally only a misdemeanor offense, such a violation may have serious repercussions, such as loss of Medicare participation and an adverse effect on credentialing by hospitals and health care plans. Moreover, professional liability insurance policies are often state-specific, so that radiologists who provide negligent advice by e-mail to patients residing in other states may find themselves without liability coverage in the event of a malpractice action.[12]

E-mail raises a host of confidentiality and security issues. Unencrypted e-mail messages can be read by third parties as easily as postcards. E-mails (as well as fax transmittals and telephone voicemail messages) can be forwarded to unintended or unknown recipients. E-mail (and fax transmittals) also can be printed out, copied, and circulated manually. Internet-based e-mail systems do not provide confirmation that a message was delivered. Even if the software is capable of indicating that the e-mail was received, it cannot ensure that the message was actually read and understood by the intended recipient. E-mail (and voicemail) rely on a central computer platform, which not only stores and forwards the message but also can restore it even after an individual user deletes it. Although deleting an e-mail removes the message from the screen and hard drive of an individual terminal, the record of the e-mail is not permanently deleted.[13]

Because of privacy concerns, radiologists and other physicians who use e-mail must take reasonable precautions to prevent patient-related e-mail from being exposed to unauthorized entry. "Encryption software can act as a type of envelope, scrambling the message contents until they are received by the intended addressee, and can provide a guarantee of a message's authenticity and integrity." Nevertheless, radiologists should recognize the problem of sending encrypted messages to patients at their workplace e-mail addresses, where they may be viewed by their employers. Radiologists face a similar problem if they use e-mail provided by their employers. Of even greater concern, "physicians who are employed by state public health agencies and other governmental bodies may find that their e-mail messages are subject to public record laws; accordingly, such practitioners must take additional steps to omit identifying patient data in e-mail messages." Consequently, radiologists must "take precautions to avoid inadvertent forwarding, copying, and printing of e-mail that would otherwise further expose patient confidences."[14]

As a part of the medical record that provides direct evidence of a patient-physician conversation, e-mail communications should be stored electronically or printed in hardcopy and placed in the patient's permanent file. As noted above, deleting e-mail messages is of little value, since they are both recoverable and legally discoverable. Because of possible violations of privacy, patients should be informed of the potential risks and benefits of using e-mail. It may be prudent to obtain a full written consent after explaining the degree of access to the patient's file by others and the security measures that are in place. "Because e-mail messages may be stored and read by employers, patients should be reminded that particularly sensitive medical information should not be sent through office e-mail even with encryption.... [Moreover,] patients must be given an opportunity to expressly prohibit identifiable, medically related communication from appearing in e-mail.[15]

Radiologists who have Web sites should be careful about providing links to other sites, since this may imply endorsement of the service, information, or products found of the linked site. "This is especially problematic because a Web site can be constantly altered and updated, making monitoring of it very difficult. Although courts have not evaluated link liability, a recent proposal for adding a 'hyperlink disclaimer' might offer some protection. Such a disclaimer would explain that the provision of links does not imply an endorsement of the information or products offered through the linked sites." Links to hospitals or health plans that provide only information to that particular entity may run afoul of antitrust, anti-kickback, and anti-self-referral statutes. Statements claiming that medical advice or second opinions rendered via the Internet do not constitute the practice of medicine have not yet been tested for their legal effect, though in previous contexts such disclaimers have rarely insulated practitioners from the prevailing standards of care.[16]

Endnotes

1 Smith JJ, Berlin L. E-mail consultation. *AJR* 2002;179:1133–1136.

2 *Reynolds v Decatur Memorial Hospital*, 277 3d80 (Ill App 1996).

3 *Clanton v Von Haam*, 340 SE2d 627 (Ga App 1986).

4 Smith JJ, Berlin L. E-mail consultation. *AJR* 2002;179:1133–1136.

5 Kuszler PC. Telemedicine and integrated health care delivery: compounding malpractice liability. *Am J Law Med* 1999;25:297–326.

6 Berlin L. Curbstone consultations. *AJR* 2002;178:1353–1359.

7 Smith JJ, Berlin L. E-mail consultation. *AJR* 2002;179:1133–1136.

8 Ibid.

9 Eysenbach G, Diepgen TL. Responses to unsolicited patient e-mail requests for medical advice on the World Wide Web. *JAMA* 1998;280:1333–1336.

10 Wakelin S, Oliver CW. How should orthopaedic surgeons respond to unsolicited e-mail? *J Bone Joint Surg [Br]* 2001;83B:482–485.

11 Spielberg AR. Online without a net: physician-patient communication by electronic mail. *Am J Law Med Ethics* 1999;25:267–295.

12 Smith JJ, Zibners H. Legal issues and formal policies. In: Dreyer KJ, Mehta A, Thrall JH, eds. *PACS: A Guide to the Digital Revolution*. New York: Springer-Verlag 2002:351–373.

13 Spielberg AR. Online without a net: physician-patient communication by electronic mail. *Am J Law Med Ethics* 1999;25:267–295.

14 Spielberg AR. On call and online: sociohistorical, legal, and ethical implications of e-mail for the patient-physician relationship. *JAMA* 1998;280:1353–1359.

15 Ibid.

16 Ibid.

33
Picture Archiving and Communications Systems (PACS)

The explosive growth of PACS technology, which has become an integral component of many radiology practices, has easily outpaced the development of laws related to the production, storage, and transmission of these digital images. Although federal and some state laws have begun to regulate computerized and electronically stored images,[1] there is no case law that specifically addresses these topics. Consequently, it is necessary to infer what courts will decide based on previous rulings that can be analogized to the PACS environment.

Data generated from PACS activities are medical records. As such, the rules developed for maintaining and storing film and paper records should serve as an appropriate guide for handling them, though by their very nature electronic data will require some special considerations. Because of the huge amount of data generated in electronic medical images and the amount of storage necessary to archive them, many facilities compress data to save costs. This should present no problem as long as reversible compression is utilized. However, the use of irreversible ("lossy") compression raises the potential of a medical record being altered and clinically relevant data being lost.[2] This can have devastating consequences if the lost images are required as evidence in a malpractice action. If medical records, including radiologic images, are destroyed, misplaced, or unavailable at trial, the judge may permit the jury to infer that the records would have been unfavorable to the party responsible for their safekeeping. Even the allegation that a defendant-radiologist lost a patient's PACS images could be perceived by a jury as deceit or fraud, resulting in a radiologist's being deemed liable for malpractice despite any concrete evidence supporting this decision.[3]

The retention period of medical records, which is subject to federal, state, and institutional laws and policies, should apply equally to records in an electronic format. When electronic data are acquired in one state and stored at another, it is unclear whether these data must be maintained at the transmitting site, the receiving site, or at both locations. Although the American College of Radiology (ACR) Standard for Teleradiology requires that the data must only be maintained at the transmitting site, it would seem prudent that teleradiology data being stored at the receiving facility meet the same standards as those at the transmitting institution.[4]

Maintaining strict confidentiality of stored electronic records is another potential problem, since this form of record keeping may be inherently more vulnerable to security breeches. Therefore, physicians and institutions using PACS or teleradiology have a duty to develop policies that ensure reasonable confidentiality of patients' electronically stored records.[5]

Failure to Interpret "Lost" PACS Images

At times, digitally acquired images may be obtained but not appropriately transmitted to the PACS system and thus not interpreted. This situation most commonly occurs when radiology department personnel manually enter an incorrect patient name or identification number, resulting in a mismatch between identifiers entered at the specific modality and identifiers stored in the PACS or hospital/radiology information system (HIS/RIS). This leads to a "lost study" problem in the PACS, which cannot automatically match new images with requests for old studies, or route images to appropriate work lists or stations for reporting. If such a discrepancy occurs, the PACS must either reject the images or send them to a special list for manual intervention.[6] This typically results in the PACS system generating an "uninterpreted-case" list, which must be resolved promptly. Because individual radiologists are far too busy to attend properly to such cases, it is essential either that dedicated personnel be assigned to the task or, far preferably, that there be an effective automated system to do so (as is now available in most commercial PACS systems). If an entire study or key images are lost, or if images cannot otherwise be interpreted, a member of the radiology department should promptly contact the referring physician or the patient to schedule a repeat study.[7]

Who is responsible if a failure to interpret a lost or misplaced PACS image results in patient injury? By analogy to case law dealing with more traditional forms of image interpretation, liability would probably be placed squarely (and perhaps unfairly!) on the radiologist. A radiologist who is on duty at an imaging facility effectively has agreed to interpret every radiologic study obtained during a given period. This creates a valid physician-patient relationship with every patient undergoing an imaging study. Consequently, the radiologist has a duty to interpret all such examinations in a timely fashion. Courts would probably construe the presence of patient data within a radiology information system as constituting sufficient notice to the radiologist that there was an examination that needed to be read. Failure to appreciate the existence of such a study requiring prompt interpretation could well be considered negligent conduct.[8]

It would seem counterintuitive to impose legal liability on a radiologist simply because PACS images have been lost or misplaced, especially when this relates to an error made by radiology department personnel who are employed by the hospital and over whom the radiologist has no authority. However, there is extensive case law indicating that radiologists would be liable for the actions of hospital personnel under their direct supervision, based on the doctrines of vicarious liability and the borrowed servant (see pages 22–24).[9]

Endnotes

1 Brenner RJ, Westenberg L. Film management and custody: current and future medicolegal issues. *AJR* 1996;167:1371–1375.
2 Smith JJ, Zibners H. Legal issues and formal policies. In: Dreyer KJ, Mehta A, Thrall JH, eds. *PACS: A Guide to the Digital Revolution*. New York: Springer, 2002:351–373.
3 Smith JJ, Berlin L. Picture archiving and communication systems (PACS) and the loss of patient examination records. *AJR* 2001;176:1381–1384.
4 Smith JJ, Zibners H. Legal issues and formal policies. In: Dreyer KJ, Mehta A, Thrall JH, eds. *PACS: A Guide to the Digital Revolution*. New York: Springer, 2002:351–373.
5 Ibid.
6 Clunie DA, Carrino JA. DICOM. In: Dreyer KJ, Mehta A, Thrall JH, eds. *PACS: A Guide to the Digital Revolution*. New York: Springer, 2002:73–119.
7 Smith JJ, Berlin L. Picture archiving and communication systems (PACS) and the loss of patient examination records. *AJR* 2001;176:1381–1384.
8 Ibid.
9 Ibid.

Part VI
Governmental/Regulatory

34
Credentialing and Peer Review

The landmark case of *Darling v. Charleston Community Memorial Hospital* established the principle that a hospital may be held liable for a patient injured by a staff physician, based on the theory that the hospital should have known of the physician's poor performance or incompetence but failed to investigate or take reasonable corrective actions.[1] No longer able to deny responsibility for acts and omissions of its staff physicians, hospitals developed tighter procedures for credentialing the medical staff to maintain quality patient care. In this ongoing process, each physician's training, skill, experience, and clinical competence are evaluated to ensure that the privileges granted match the level of expertise. All new applicants for privileges (or additional privileges), as well as physicians returning to practice after a significant absence, usually require proctoring. This is designed to ensure that the physician is competent to perform the procedure(s) for which privileges are requested. To encourage more aggressive peer review by medical staffs, many states have enacted immunity statutes to protect hospital peer review committees as long as they provide due process to the affected physician.[2] Federal law related to Medicare and Medicaid programs mandate some form of peer review if hospitals are to be compensated for services.[3] The Joint Committee on Accreditation of Healthcare Organizations (JCAHO) also requires that its member hospitals have a credentialing process in place to qualify for accreditation and holds the hospital's governing board ultimately responsible for peer review by its medical staff.[4]

Due Process

All physicians who first apply for privileges—or who reapply for privileges that were involuntarily restricted, suspended, or revoked—must be treated in a fair and consistent manner. After some cases of medical staff members abusing their power for discriminatory or other improper motives, state courts and legislatures have gradually extended legal protection to physicians whose staff privileges are attacked. In the past half century, the trend has been to recognize the "fundamental" right of physicians to fully practice their professions. To protect the legal rights of physicians and to protect their careers, each hospital must develop and implement clearly written due process procedures.[5]

At a minimum, due process and fair procedures include adequate notice of the charges on which any adverse action is based and the opportunity to present evidence on one's own behalf to an unbiased decision maker. However, other protections usually found in civil and criminal cases—such as the rights to be represented by counsel and cross-examine witnesses—have generally not been provided in disciplinary hearings. Most state laws allow a physician to challenge a decision restricting or terminating medical staff privileges. Although usually the physician is then limited to a review of the written record of the peer review body, occasionally courts may permit a full evidentiary hearing *de novo*. Nevertheless, courts traditionally defer to the decisions of administrative bodies (such as hospital boards and committees) and are unwilling to interfere in what is deemed the exclusive domain of hospitals and physicians.[6]

In California and some other states, courts have extended the same protections to physicians in cases involving private insurers, health maintenance organizations, and managed care payers—entities that control "important economic interests" and thus are prohibited from arbitrarily depriving a physician of privileges or contract rights without a fair hearing procedure.[7] For example, in the seminal *Delta Dental* case,[8] the fact that the plan was "the largest dental health plan in California covering over 8 million individuals" convinced the court that the managed care organization had a duty to give its member dentists the common law right to fair procedure when they challenged a reduction in payment rates. A subsequent ruling extended this right, striking down the removal of a physician from a provider network for reasons that are "arbitrary, capricious, and/or contrary to public policy," even if the contract has a termination-at-will clause.[9]

Despite the state- and court-imposed protections noted above, there are situations when a physician's medical staff privileges may be revoked or withdrawn without any recourse to due process safeguards. One is when a hospital acts for purely business or economic reasons, or for any other cause that does not relate to the physician's quality of care or fitness to practice. Thus, a hospital may close its staff or a particular service (such as radiology or anesthesiology) or award an exclusive contract to one physician or group while excluding all others (including those already on staff). Although occasionally challenged on both due process and antitrust theories, such actions have been upheld by courts ruling that hospitals have the discretion to make such decisions, even when they limit competition or damage the interests of individual physicians.[10]

Peer Review

In the late 1980s, a physician-plaintiff prevailed in a lawsuit against a group of physicians who had participated in a peer review committee that had acted to preserve their own economic interests by excluding the physician from a hospital's medical staff.[11] The multimillion-dollar verdict against the peer reviewers destroyed the community's only multispecialty practice and received national attention. Following this case, physicians were understandably reluctant to participate in peer review, thus decreasing the ability of hospitals to monitor quality of care. In response, Congress passed the Health Care Quality Improvement Act (HCQIA), which provided near-total legal protection of peer reviewers as well as creating the National Practitioner's Data Bank (see page 68).[12]

The virtual immunity of peer reviewers has had unintended consequences. Physicians whose professional lives are damaged as a result of peer review actions have extremely limited recourse, even if the review was conducted with faulty procedures or for improper reasons. Federal court decisions[13] ordering unsuccessful physician-plaintiffs to pay the attorney fees of defendant peer review members have sent a strong warning to practitioners and their legal counsel who are considering challenging a credentialing action. Rather than its original intent of evaluating physician activities and providing constructive corrective measures to help one's colleagues and improve and assure quality of care, peer review increasingly has become a punitive process for recommending limitations of clinical privileges, including the expulsion of physicians from the hospital or managed-care panel. This exclusionary power creates great risk for abuse. Because the reviewers are frequently in the same specialty, they may stand to gain financially by adversely evaluating a competing physician.[14]

Records of peer review actions and proceedings are generally exempted from discovery and may not be used as evidence in a civil suit. Medical staff bylaws often require that members hold in strict confidence all information and records relating to a peer review proceeding, lest they themselves be subjected to disciplinary action.[15]

Despite the growing trend toward protecting physicians' fundamental rights and interests in medical staff privileges, medical staffs continue to operate as autonomous entities when determining which physicians are competent to be granted credentials and which should lose them. As a peer review body, the medical staff is responsible for protecting patients from incompetent or unstable physicians. However, by improperly denying a physician access to patients and facilities, the medical staff may severely damage a physician's professional reputation, standing, and even license to practice medicine. At every stage in the peer review process, the affected physician is at a disadvantage. A disciplinary hearing operating under medical staff bylaws is like a malpractice action, but with the colleagues of the accused physician acting as witnesses, prosecutors, and judges. There is little opportunity to obtain discovery of evidence before it is presented. Hearsay evidence is permitted, including the medical opinions of experts who cannot be compelled to appear and be cross-examined. The accused physician may be denied the right to the assistance of counsel and to subpoena witnesses and documents, and witnesses in a peer review hearing may enjoy absolute immunity from civil suits for slander or malicious injury, even if their testimony is false. The hospital and medical staff members are also immune from suit under federal law unless it is proved that they acted in bad faith when taking the peer review action. Because the consequences of a decision adversely affecting medical staff privileges are so severe¾including mandatory reporting by the hospital to the state medical board and National Practitioners Data Bank, which is accessible to hospitals and managed-care organizations¾there have been calls to extend procedural due process principles to all facets of the peer review process.[16]

Endnotes

1 *Darling v Charleston Community Memorial Hospital*, 211 N.E.2d 253, 260 (1965).
2 Firestone M, Schur RE. Medical staff peer rebview in the credentialing and privileging of physicians. In: Sanbar SS, Gibofsky A, Firestone MH, et al (eds). *Legal Medicine, 5th ed*. St. Louis, Mosby, 2001, pg., 78.
3 Blum. Medical peer review. 38 *J Legal Educ*. 525 at 531 (1988).
4 Firestone M, Schur RE. Medical staff peer rebview in the credentialing and privileging of physicians. In: Sanbar SS, Gibofsky A, Firestone MH, et al (eds). *Legal Medicine, 5th ed*. St. Louis, Mosby, 2001, pg., 78.
5 Ibid., 79.
6 Ibid., 79–81.
7 Ibid., 79.
8 *Delta Dental Plan of California v Banasky*, 33 Cal. Rptr. 2d 381 (Cal App 1994).

9 *Ambrosino v Metropolitan Life Insurance Comp*any, 899 F.Supp 438 (N.D. Cal 1995).

10 Firestone M, Schur RE. Medical staff peer rebview in the credentialing and privileging of physicians. In: Sanbar SS, Gibofsky A, Firestone MH, et al (eds). *Legal Medicine, 5th ed*. St. Louis, Mosby, 2001, pg., 81.

11 *Patrick v Burget*, 486 U.S. 94 (1988).

12 Livingston EH, Harwell JD. Peer review. *Am J Surg* 2001;182:103–109.

13 *Smith v Ricks*, 31 F3d 1478, 1489 (9th Cir 1994).

14 Livingston EH, Harwell JD. Peer review. *Am J Su*rg 2001;182:103–109.

15 Firestone M, Schur RE. Medical staff peer rebview in the credentialing and privileging of physicians. In: Sanbar SS, Gibofsky A, Firestone MH, et al (eds). *Legal Medicine, 5th ed*. St. Louis, Mosby, 2001, pg., 81.

16 Ibid., 81–82.

35
Infected or Substance-Abuse-Impaired Radiologist[1]

Radiologists who suffer from certain physical conditions may pose a potential risk to their patients. This problem has been exacerbated in recent years with the increase in radiologists who have a transmissible blood-borne disease or who are impaired by substance abuse. In addition to the direct liability of the infected or impaired radiologist whose conduct leads to patient injury, the radiology group or hospital may also be liable if it knew or should have known of the radiologist's condition. A related issue is whether a radiologist's infected or impaired status must be disclosed as part of the informed consent process.

Liability of the Infected/Impaired Radiologist

Since the days of Hippocrates, physicians have recognized an ethical duty to avoid injuring the patients they treat. As the Code of Medical Ethics of the American Medical Association explicitly states,[2] "It is unethical for a physician to practice medicine while under the influence of a controlled substance, alcohol, or other chemical agents which impair the ability to practice medicine." Furthermore, "a physician who knows that he or she is seropositive should not engage in any activity that creates a significant risk of transmission of that disease to a patient." In addition to moral concerns, courts in malpractice lawsuits have held that the actual transmission of an infectious agent from physician to patient may violate the standard of care. Needle-stick injuries in the health care setting have been shown to result in nosocomial viral transmission, which is estimated to occur after needle sticks in 3% for hepatitis C, 30% for hepatitis B, and 0.3% for HIV.[3]

Violation of the standard of care is virtually certain when an impaired radiologist's direct actions or inaccurate diagnosis causes harm to a patient, or when there has been actual transmission of an infectious disease between radiologist and patient. Moreover, in the case of an infected physician, the courts have recognized patient injury even in the absence of actual disease transmission. A patient who has been subjected to an invasive procedure may be awarded compensation after the mere exposure to the bodily fluids of an infected provider, or even because of the reasonable fear of infection when the patient subsequently discovers that the physician performing the procedure had a potentially transmissible disease. One court referred to studies indicating that a surgeon cuts a glove in about one in four cases and sustains a significant skin cut in one out of forty cases; although the risk of infection from surgeon to patient is unlikely, "there does come a point where the risk of a detrimental outcome becomes sufficiently real."[4] In another case, even though a patient did not test positive for HIV virus after a procedure performed by an HIV-infected surgeon, a court awarded compensation for such injuries as "fear and mental and emotional distress ... accompanied by headache, sleeplessness, and the physical and financial sting of blood tests for the AIDS virus."[5]

Consequently, as Berlin has observed, "An infected or substance abuse-impaired radiologist who is aware of his or her condition must take all reasonable steps to minimize any potential for patient injury and should not engage in any activity that creates a significant risk of injury or transmission of disease to a patient."

Liability of Other Parties

A radiology group or hospital that is aware or should be aware ("actual or presumptive knowledge") that an infected or impaired radiologist poses a potential risk to patients may be legally liable for the harm caused to patients by that radiologist. Actual knowledge would exist if an infected radiologist reported his or her condition to the department chairman or major hospital official, or if these individuals received witnessed incidents of substance abuse or its effects. Conversely, it is unlikely that a court would hold that a radiology group or hospital should have been aware of an infected radiologist who was asymptomatic and did not reveal his condition. The courts have been extremely reluctant to allow mandatory testing of hospital staff, unless there is a strong showing of likely infection and reasonable concern of its transmission to patients. If a physician shows even a suggestion of substance abuse, some courts have indicated that the department chair or hospital should take appropriate action, rather than waiting until a patient is injured or killed.[6] Conceivably, this could be extended to making mandatory testing a condition of employment, even when there are only relatively subtle or equivocal signs of drug or alcohol abuse.

Once a radiology group or hospital has knowledge or suspects that a radiologist suffers from substance abuse or is infected with a potentially transmissible disease, it is essential that steps be taken immediately to prevent any possible danger to patients. For infected radiologists, this may require being prohibited from performing biopsies, angiography, and other interventional procedures so as to eliminate the risk of transmission of the infection to patients.

Informed Consent

Based on a duty to warn, the courts have ruled that informing a patient of a radiologist's potentially transmissible disease may be required as part of the informed consent process. The situation is not as clear with substance abuse, though a strong dissent in one court observed that in a physician-patient relationship, "Silence when one should speak or failure to disclose what one ought to reveal is equivalent to an actual false misrepresentation.... Consent which is obtained by a material misrepresentation is invalid, since fraud vitiates all contracts."[7] If the patient has relied on a material misrepresentation and sustained injury, the physician could be liable for battery, unlike the usual malpractice case based on negligence or breaching the standard of care. This could allow the plaintiff to succeed at trial without showing that the physician deviated from the appropriate standard of care, as well as expose the physician to punitive damages and damages for "mental anguish resulting from the belated knowledge that the operation was performed by a doctor whom the patient had [without being informed of the physician's condition] given consent."[8]

Therefore, Berlin concludes that when "a radiologist with a known substance-abuse impairment or potentially transmissible disease is involved in radiologic procedures that may result in disease transmission or other patient injury, consideration should be given to including information about the impairment or infection as part of the informed consent process."

Endnotes

1 Smith JJ, Berlin L. The infected or substance abuse-impaired radiologist. *AJR* 2002;178:567–571.

2 American Medical Association Council on Ethical and Judicial Affairs. Principles of medical ethics. In: *Code of Medical Ethics: Current Opinions with Annotations*. Chicago: American Medical Association 2000;188:222–224.

3 Lauer GM, Walker BD. Hepatitis C virus infection. *N Engl J Med* 2001;345:41–49.

4 *Behringer v Medical Center at Princeton*, 592 A2d 1251 (NJ Super 1991).

5 *Faya v Almaraz*, 620 A2d 327 (MD App 1993).
6 *Babcock v St. Francis Medical Center*, 543 NW2d 749 (Neb App 1996).
7 *Bekker v Humana Health Plan*, Inc. 229 F3d 662 (7th Cir US App 2000).
8 *Howard v Univ of Med and Dentistry of New Jersey*, 768 A2d 195 (NJ Super 2001).

36
Federal Fraud and Abuse Enforcement and Compliance Plans[1,2]

Fraud and Abuse

According to a report of the Office of the Inspector General (OIG) of the Department of Health and Human Services (HHS), in 1996 Medicare disbursed about $23 billion in overpayments for inappropriate and possibly fraudulent services; more than 20% of these improper payments went to physicians. The OIG estimated that spending attributable to waste, fraud, and abuse ranges from 3% to 10% of national health care expenditures. In an effort to recoup some of this huge sum, the authority of the federal government to combat health care fraud was clarified and its enforcement ability was significantly expanded with the enactment of the Health Insurance Portability and Accountability Act of 1996 (HIPAA). Among its provisions, "This law doubled the number of OIG auditors and investigators in addition to expanding the power of the Federal Bureau of Investigation to investigate health care fraud; created the Medicare Integrity Program whereby HHS may enter into contracts with private entities to review and audit activities where Medicare provides coverage; and established a reward program to encourage Medicare beneficiaries to report questionable behavior." Consequently, physicians submitting a claim for payment must be aware that the federal government has the authority to investigate its propriety. An inappropriate claim for payment, ranging from an inadvertent mistake to outright fraud, may lead to liability to both criminal and civil sanctions (monetary fines). Civil sanctions, which require that the physician "knew or should have known" that a claim was inaccurate or prohibited, may be as much as $10,000 per claim ($50,000 for an anti-kickback violation) plus an assessment of up to three times the amount improperly claimed. Criminal penalties may be imposed where an individual "knowingly and willfully" defrauds the Medicare, Medicaid, or other federal health care benefits program. The fraudulent submission of even a single claim may result in "imprisonment for up to five years; a fine of up $250,000 per claim; and a five-year exclusion (lifetime exclusion for a third conviction) from participation in the Medicare and Medicaid programs."

An important feature of the federal False Claims Act is its "*qui tam*" ("whistle-blower") provision. This enables private citizens (or organizations) to earn substantial amounts of money by bringing a false claims action against a radiologist or other health care provider on behalf of the United States government. The *qui tam* provision is a powerful financial incentive for private entities to pursue a Medicare fraud and abuse action, since the resulting awards can range from 10% to 30% of the settlement or judgment (depending on whether the government chooses of become a part of the action). The only limitation on a *qui tam* action is that the entity making the accusation must be the "original source" of the information (i.e., have had "direct and independent knowledge"); it is not sufficient if the person or organization merely learned of potentially fraudulent behavior from a public source and then filed a suit.

It is fraud for radiologists to bill for services that were not performed. However, it is similarly fraudulent to bill for services that were performed by another health care provider (such as a nurse or technologist) who is not eligible to bill under Medicate Part B "without the supervision or active participation of the billing radiologist." The situation is especially complicated in academic institutions with accredited radiology resident programs. As "trainees," the financial support for residents comes in part through Medicare Part A payments made to their institutions. Because the government has deemed this as payment for the residents' services to Medicare beneficiaries, they are not eligible also to bill Medicare Part B for any services provided to such patients as part of their training program. Attending radiologists supervising radiology residents in a teaching setting may bill Medicare Part B, but only for services that they "personally" render to beneficiaries. According to the federal rules, this means that the attending radiologist must be present during "key" or "critical" portions of the resident-provided service or procedure. For diagnostic radiology, this requires that the teaching radiologist either personally interpret the study or actually review the resident's interpretation (not merely countersigning an official report). For interventional procedures, the attending radiologist must be physically present during all "critical portions" (not precisely defined) of the procedure and be immediately available during the entire procedure. In recent years, the federal government has been increasingly aggressive in enforcing these Medicare billing regulations through Physicians at Teaching Hospitals (PATH) audits. These have resulted in large negotiated settlements by training institutions that have been accused of not adhering to the fraud and abuse guidelines.

"Moonlighting" residents who provide services to Medicare beneficiaries outside the scope of their formal training programs may bill Medicare for Part B payments.

Compliance Plans

Radiologists and other health care professionals should be proactive in meeting the new federal fraud enforcement guidelines by establishing a compliance plan. The existence of an effective compliance plan provides evidence that any mistakes were inadvertent (i.e., no intent to commit an illegal act) and is one significant factor that both the OIG and the Department of Justice will take into account "in determining whether a medical practice or other health care entity has made reasonable efforts to avoid and detect misbehavior" and "in determining the level of sanctions, penalties, and exclusions that may be sought and imposed." While the development of an effective compliance plan entails some cost, this is outweighed by the advantages of "identifying under- and over-coding; reducing the likelihood of civil or criminal wrongdoing; and reducing potential penalties if wrongdoing is detected."

Although an effective compliance plan must be specifically tailored to fit the individual organization and its operation, it should contain the following seven basic elements:

a. Commitment to compliance
b. Designation of a compliance officer
c. Routine training and education programs
d. Auditing and monitoring
e. Effective lines of communication
f. Internal investigation and disciplinary processes
g. Response to offenses and ability to take corrective action

Commitment to Compliance

Everyone in the organization must understand the necessity to comply with established standards and the fact that the organization will take actions to uphold these standards. The organization (management, board of directors, partners, owner) must accept the duty of compliance and commit resources sufficient to identify and prevent any criminal conduct.

Designation of a Compliance Officer

The compliance officer must be a trustworthy individual who holds a high level of responsibility for setting policy and has the ability to influence behavior and organizational practices. He or she must have sufficient authority to administer the compliance plan effectively; typically, this means that the individual will report directly to the highest levels of management. The compliance officer may delegate authority to other trustworthy individuals. Background checks may be required for new employees who will be involved in activities where compliance questions are addressed, such as billing and coding activities.

Routine Training and Education Programs

The organization must have a routine training and education process that includes an overview of the laws relating to fraud and abuse, the operation and importance of the compliance plan, and the role of each employee in it. Under the direction of the compliance officer and using a variety of techniques and materials, these educational activities must be conducted on a regular (at least annual) basis, with the frequency of participation dictated by an individual's function in the organization. Those directly involved in areas with a significant potential for health care fraud and abuse require more extensive training commensurate with their individual responsibilities. For example, physicians need to understand their responsibility to document the care provided in the medical record so that it conforms to billing requests. The organization should maintain a record of both its training activities and individual participation in them.

Auditing and Monitoring

A key action demonstrating a commitment to compliance is the implementation of an effective system of auditing and monitoring the practices of the organization. There must be a regular review of the process from the moment when a service for a patient is initiated to the submission of a claim for payment, including the mechanism for employee reporting of suspected situations of fraud or abuse.

The audit process should be utilized to (a) establish a baseline in initiating a compliance plan; (b) periodically assess the effectiveness of the organization; (c) monitor the work of new employees; and (d) respond to complaints. "The baseline audit should examine the claim development and submission process ... and identify elements within this process that may contribute to non-compliance or that may need to be the focus for improving execution. This audit should establish a consistent methodology for selecting and examining records" that will be utilized in future audits. The baseline audit may be conducted based on claims submitted during the initial three months after the education and training program. Subsequently, periodic audits need to be conducted on at least an annual cycle, though quarterly audits are recommended. "The goal of these audits should be to assure personnel competency and uncover improper claims activity (especially patterns of improper activity) prior to the point where potential violations may be significant enough that the government would impose penalties. An effective periodic audit process must include a means to provide feedback to individuals involved in the various phases of claim development and submission."

In addition to participating in education and training activities, new employees must have their work monitored to ensure that it is consistent with the standards to prevent fraud and abuse. Where new employees are involved in the claims process (from development to submission), at least a sample of the claims they have handled should be audited until the compliance officer is satisfied with the individual's level of competence. In addition to its employees, the organization may be responsible for the activities of individuals who provide services for the organization, such as independent contractors.

Organizations must be prepared to conduct audits in response to complaints from employees or patients, or in the face of other evidence of possible improper billing practices. Failure to respond promptly to a complaint raises questions as to an organization's commitment to compliance. Complaints must be taken seriously, and individuals need to understand that they may make complaints without fear of retribution.

Effective Lines of Communication

Communications must be able to flow in both directions between the compliance officer and professional and support personnel within the organization. Effective communication is a two-way process that must involve all parties in an organization. The compliance officer must be able to provide information about the organization's standards and the results of audit and other compliance information, and individuals employed by or otherwise involved with the organization must be able to communicate questions and complaints to the compliance officer.

A "hotline" should be established to facilitate the reporting of suspected violations. Any person using this process should be confident that his or her confidentiality will be maintained, there will be no retaliation, and each complaint will be investigated thoroughly.

Internal Investigation and Disciplinary Processes

When there is information of potential violations or misconduct, the chief compliance officer (or designee) has the responsibility of conducting an internal investigation that includes interviews and a review of the medical record, billing forms, and other relevant documents. "To assure protection from coerced disclosure for information gained through investigative interviews, statistical and record analyses and other reports, consideration should be given to having the investigation conducted by qualified legal counsel. The attorney/client privilege will afford a level of protection in the event that the OIG or another agency requests information developed in the course of an internal investigation."

Disciplinary measures must be applied fairly. This requires that the organization maintain a written internal enforcement and discipline policy and keep records whenever it is applied.

Response to Offenses and Corrective Action

When a compliance problem has been identified, the organization has a responsibility to take demonstrable corrective actions, including steps to prevent further similar offenses. When there has been the receipt of overpayments or other deviations from federal legal standards, corrective action (including repayment as appropriate) should be initiated. A difficult question (which should be discussed with legal counsel) is whether an organization should voluntarily disclose compliance problems to the federal government. This is not mandatory and does not provide any automatic protections or guarantees of leniency. "In considering whether to report a detected offense, it must be noted that OIG enforcement investigations may be initiated based on carrier records, a call from a disgruntled employee, a patient complaint, and even an anonymous tip to the HHS Confidential Tip Line. In the event that an internal investigation discovers that a material violation has occurred, it sometimes may be advisable to report the matter to the federal government." However, since "failure to disclose will call into question the veracity of the plan and limit the reduced culpability protections that the plan is designed to afford, disclosure may be appropriate."

Documentation

Documentation is a central component of an effective compliance plan. In addition to facilitating quality patient care, accurate patient records are valuable legal documents for providing the justification necessary to support claims payment. "The medical record may be used to validate the site or the medical service, the medical necessity and appropriateness of diagnostic and/or therapeutic services provided, and that the services have been reported accurately." The reason for ordering diagnostic and other ancillary services should be explicitly stated or easily inferred, and the CPT (Current Procedural Terminology) and ICD-9-CM (International Classification of Diseases) codes reported on the health insurance claim form should be supported by documentation in the medical record.

Endnotes

1 American Medical Association at: *www.ama-assn.org.*

2 Smith JJ, Berlin B. Medicare fraud and abuse. *AJR* 2003;180:591–595.

37
Professional Courtesy[1,2]

Professional courtesy refers to taking care of other physicians or their families free of charge or at a reduced rate. A long-standing tradition in the medical profession dating back to Hippocrates, the practice has served to build bonds between physicians and to reduce the incentive for physicians to treat their own families. However, in recent years Congress and private insurance companies have greatly reduced the permissible scope for reducing charges for medical care. Physicians who do not adhere to these rules may be violating a variety of federal and state laws and risk denial of claims and even de-selection from the managed health plans. Private insurers and the federal government have basic restrictions on how a physician charges patients for medical care, and neither creates an exception for professional courtesy. In general, if physicians cannot reduce the cost of care for anyone else in their practices, they cannot reduce it for other physicians. Moreover, there are even situations where it is permissible to reduce the cost of care for everyone *except* physicians.

The most common way for a physician to reduce the cost of care for patients is to waive the co-payment. Many insurers impose co-payments for office visits and other medical services to make patients more conscious of the cost of their medical care and to discourage unnecessary visits to health providers. The theory is that forcing the patient to share the cost of treatment will create a more sophisticated health care consumer. However, the reality is that the co-payment limits access to care for many people, which translates into less money that the health plan has to pay to physicians and hospitals for that care.

In most situations, both private insurers and the federal government ban waiving the co-payment (though Medicare has some provisions allowing it to be waived in documented cases of financial hardship) and require the physician to make reasonable efforts to collect co-payments that are billed to the patient. The routine waiver of co-payments has been construed as a fraudulent misrepresentation of physician charges against payers of all types. For example, physicians have often characterized professional courtesy as accepting whatever the insurance plan allows as payment in full. However, when the patient is a Medicare beneficiary, such an action can have serious repercussions. Under traditional Medicare, physicians are paid 80% of the allowable amount—the payment schedule amount or the actual charge, whichever is lower. As an example, if Medicare allows $100 for a certain procedure, the program pays $80 and the co-payment amount is $20. If the physician adopts the policy of accepting only "what insurance pays" as payment in full, this could be construed as implying that the actual charge was $80, so that the resulting insurance payment should be only $64. If the physician files a claim listing a usual and customary fee of $100, this could be considered as a misrepresentation of the fee to the plan (i.e., accepting a new total fee for the rendering of the service but billing the insurer the regular fee). The routine promise to waive co-payments also can be deemed as an unfair trade practice, since it allows the billing of third-party payers for more than the health care provider was willing to accept and prevents others from competing unless they adopted similar fraudulent practices.

Another approach is for a physician to offer a "discount." However, many private insurance plans and some federal programs have a "most favored nation" clause in physician contracts, which entitles the plan to pay the lowest charge the physician bills to anyone. Any systematic pattern of discounts could trigger a reduction in the physician's allowable reimbursement schedule to the discounted price.

Extending professional courtesy by offering free care could be viewed as a violation of the federal anti-kickback law if there is a link between the care provided and subsequent referral of patients who are Medicare or Medicaid beneficiaries. Any payment or inducement that might tend to affect referral decisions is prohibited, even if it has another valid purpose. For example, a surgeon who only gave professional courtesy to physicians who referred him business would clearly violate the law. Professional courtesy based on being on the same hospital staff would raise the same issues, although the link to referrals is more tenuous. Giving professional courtesy to all physicians without conditions would be more defensible, but if the government could show that a disproportionate number of physicians receiving the courtesy were also referring physicians, a court might well rule that this was a prohibited inducement.

Traditionally, if physicians violated the terms of their contracts with private insurers, the insurer could refuse to pay the claim, de-select the physician from the plan, and even sue the physician for fraud. The Health

Insurance Portability and Accountability Act of 1996 (HIPAA), better known as the Kennedy-Kassebaum bill, now makes it a federal crime to defraud private insurance companies and could result in stiff fines and criminal prosecution. The federal government can also refuse to pay the claim and has the power to ban the physician from participation in Medicare and Medicaid. Although there have been no reported cases, prosecutions, or settlements related to this issue, physicians who offer professional courtesy should be absolutely certain that this is not linked to referrals, either in reality or in appeaance.

Endnotes

1 Rathbun KC, Richards EP III. Professional courtesy. *Missouri Med* 1998;95:18–20.
2 American Medical Association at: *www.ama-assn.org*.

38
Sexual Harassment[1]

Sexual harassment violates Title VII of the 1964 Civil Rights Act, a comprehensive piece of legislation that prohibits discrimination based on race, color, religion, sex, or national origin.

Sexual Harassment Policy

Employers should establish a written sexual harassment policy, which protects both employer and employee by defining the scope of inappropriate behavior and its consequences, as well as the responsibilities of all involved. The policy must state that sexual harassment is not only against company policy but is forbidden by law. Behaviors that constitute harassment need to be described, either in general or explicit terms. In a more detailed policy, a list of specific actions to be avoided includes "touching, pinching, and hugging; verbal presentations including sexually oriented jokes or jokes that degrade men or women; visual exhibits consisting of sexually oriented objects or displays [calendars, pin-ups, and cartoons]; and comments that promise benefits from sexual acts." There must be an indication of the appropriate method for initiating complaints and the types of remedial action available. Providing precise details in a sexual harassment policy can eliminate confusion and prevent "creative" interpretations that might occur with oral or nonspecific written policies.

The policy must provide a procedure for reporting sexual harassment. In certain circumstances, a single avenue of complaint is too confining, as when the immediate supervisor is the alleged harasser. It must be explicitly stated that the employer will punish and even terminate the employment of harassers, regardless of their rank in the organization. The policy also should state that the complainant will be protected from retaliation.

The primary goal of a sexual harassment policy is to prevent incidents, not to address and remedy problems once they occur. Consequently, some organizations have instituted programs in sensitivity training as part of their new employee orientation or as regular in-service sessions.

Allegations of Sexual Harassment

There are two basic arguments made by a person claiming that she or he has been the victim of sexual harassment. *Quid pro quo* is the term given to a situation in which submission to sexual advances is a condition of the individual's continued employment or advancement. *Hostile work environment* is sexual harassment that depends on the "totality of the circumstances" of the case, which is determined on the basis of the type(s) of behavior involved, its frequency and degree of offensiveness, and the professional relationship of the harasser and the victim. The evidence must be sufficient to convince a court that true harassment has occurred—often not an easy task. Repeated sexual innuendo or the use of vulgar gender-based epithets, as well as termination or elimination from promotion based on gender, has been considered enough to constitute a hostile work environment. Acts that are not overtly sexual but occur because of the sex of the employee may be construed as sexual harassment, as when a man threatens a woman with physical violence or verbally abuses her in the workplace. Unwelcome sexual conduct by itself is not necessarily sexual harassment. Minor degrees of gender discrimination—so-called "microinequities" ranging from unconscious or conscious slights, invisibility (making a suggestion that is overlooked until made by someone more powerful or for which someone more powerful assumes responsibility), and exploitation (making assignments so that certain people are always doing less glamorous rotations and their careers are negatively affected)—are not legally actionable.

Although in most reported cases of sexual harassment the victim is female and the harasser is male, the opposite may occur. Some cases involve male victims subjected to harassment from female supervisors. Courts have recently even addressed cases of same-sex harassment, generally quid pro quo actions by male employees against male supervisors.

What to Do If One Is a Victim of Sexual Harassment

Even if one sincerely believes that she (or he) is the victim of unwelcome sexual advances or any form of sexual harassment, it is possible that the law may not agree. The first step is to carefully review and adhere to the employer-established sexual harassment policy. It is essential to keep a careful written record by documenting those acts of harassment that have occurred and any subsequent acts of harassment or retaliation. If available, one should identify any witnesses to these events. Unless the situation is life-threatening, such as if rape or murder were a real possibility, it is not advisable to refuse to return to work until receiving assurance that the problem has been resolved, for unexcused absences may only jeopardize one's position.

A victim of alleged sexual harassment may choose to communicate her or his concerns directly to the alleged harasser. This method alone may be effective in stopping the harassment, especially if it was based merely on a misunderstanding. A written warning about the offensive behavior (with a copy to the supervisor) may alert the harasser to the seriousness of the situation and be all that is needed to end the disagreeable conduct. It also provides documentation if the case results in formal proceedings or legal action.

An individual who is subjected to sexual harassment may exercise the option of legal action, though this can take years and be extremely expensive. A claim may be filed with the federal Equal Employment Opportunity Commission (EEOC) or equivalent state agency within up to 300 days of the occurrence of the alleged sexual harassment.

Employer Course of Action

Federal law mandates prompt and complete investigation of a sexual harassment claim due to its seriousness and potential urgency. It is in the employer's best interest to pursue a vigorous investigation so as to arrive at the truth, since successful litigation following an inadequate investigation may expose the employer to punitive damages. Formal proceedings, while they may be a part of an organization's investigational policy, are not required by law. Documents from the investigation become part of the legal record and may be used as evidence in any subsequent lawsuit. However, communications between the employer and legal counsel are usually privileged and not subject to discovery.

The first step in an investigation is to objectively assess the validity of the claim. If there truly has been harassment, the employer can decide appropriate remedial or disciplinary action to promptly eliminate the circumstances that permitted the harassment to occur. If the mere presence of the harasser creates a hostile work environment, the harasser may have to be transferred or even dismissed if no suitable position is available. The harasser may have to be placed on probation, required to attend sensitivity training or perform community service, and warned that any repetition of the harassment will result in termination of employment. If the situation is not remedied or the remedy is only temporary or ineffectual, the employer can be held liable for any subsequent occurrences of harassment.

It is essential that the victim never be punished to alleviate the situation. Thus, the victim must not be transferred to a less desirable position in order to prevent a hostile work environment.

A claim of sexual harassment is deemed so serious that an employer has a legal obligation to investigate it, even if it is subsequently withdrawn by the employee. The employer must act on the initial complaint because it may be unclear whether the employee withdrew the allegation because it was groundless or due to fear of reprisal. If another person is subsequently pursued by the alleged harasser, the employer may have greater liability because of not performing a thorough investigation of the initial complaint. Moreover, the initial complainant may later decide to sue, even if previously requesting that no action be taken.

The employer must not reprimand the alleged harasser solely on the basis of claims by the alleged victim. Some sexual harassment claims are untrue and are merely attempts at revenge for real or imagined slights. An employee who has been passed over for promotion may allege that the supervisor involved and the subordinate who did receive the promotion engaged in sexual misconduct. Moreover, an alleged harasser who is subjected to disciplinary action, but ultimately cleared of any wrongdoing, may be able to pursue legal action against the employer.

Endnote

1 Feinstein KA. Sexual harassment. In: *Risk Management: Test and Syllabus*. Reston, VA: American College of Radiology, 1999:43-50.

39
Employee Retirement Income Security Act (ERISA)

As a general rule, all organizations are legally liable for causing personal injury as a result of their own negligence or the negligence of their employees and agents. However, a major exception has resulted from judicial interpretation of the Employee Retirement Income Security Act of 1974 (ERISA), which has been deemed to grant health benefit plans provided by employers or unions (and the managed-care organizations that sell or administer them) immunity from ordinary tort liability for their own negligence with respect to members of the plan.[1] ERISA was originally enacted to create comprehensive and uniform federal regulation of employee welfare and benefit plans. To ensure consistent regulations of these plans and to avoid having them caught up in the often-conflicting laws of various state and local governments, ERISA contains a preemption clause that requires it to supersede all state laws so far as they "relate to" any employee benefit plan.[2] Activities that "relate to" an ERISA plan include determining eligibility for claims, calculating and paying benefits, monitoring available funds, and keeping records.[3]

Until recently, the courts have interpreted ERISA as mandating that any lawsuit challenging the manner in which an employee benefit plan is administered, including one alleging medical malpractice, be filed within the federal court system; if the case initially was filed in a state court, the suit must be transferred ("removed") to a federal court.[4] In contrast, patients who belong to a government-sponsored health plan (such as government employees) or who buy individual health insurance policies are entitled to sue the plan or its administrators under the general state laws of tort liability. ERISA grants beneficiaries of health plans sponsored by employers and unions legal remedies for denial of benefits, but not for negligent decisions about medical treatment. A patient may sue the plan or administering managed-care organization (in federal court) to recover a wrongfully denied benefit or treatment. However, a successful claimant is entitled to recover only the dollar amount of the benefit that was denied, such as the cost of a diagnostic test or surgical procedure. Unlike in a state negligence action for medical malpractice, compensation is not permitted for loss resulting from personal injuries, such as medical expenses or lost wages, or for the death of a patient who died because of lack of treatment.[5]

Since 1995, however, a growing number of federal circuit courts have carved out an exception to the ERISA immunity by allowing managed-care organizations that serve ERISA plans to be sued in state court if the physician who provided negligent care to the patient acted as an employee or agent of the managed-care organization.[6] The underlying rationale for allowing liability in such cases is that the employee's (physician's) medical judgments are decisions that determine the quality of care and thus do not "relate to" (involve the terms of) an ERISA plan. However, few physicians are actually employees of managed-care organizations, even though they contract with a health plan to provide care to enrolled patients. Therefore, this initially left the physicians themselves as the primary target of medical malpractice claims.[7] However, subsequent cases have held that managed-care organizations can be held vicariously liable for negligent actions of independently practicing contracted physicians even if they are not direct employees.[8] This is based on a theory of *ostensible agency*—if the managed-care organization acted in a manner that would lead the "reasonable person to conclude that [her doctor] was an employee or agent.... Aggressive advertising campaigns arguably create the expectation in the public that [HMOs] are providers of health care," and this effectively assures patients of the high quality of their doctors.[9]

Several cases have claimed that managed-care organizations violate their fiduciary duty by making financial arrangements that create incentives for physicians to withhold necessary care, or by failing to disclose the existence of such incentives to plan members. In effect, this practice creates a conflict of interest that forces physicians to choose between personal profit and the health of their patients.[10] In a landmark case,[11] the Supreme Court rejected the idea that "treatment decisions" (primarily concerning medical services, not financial decisions) made by a managed-care organization, acting through its physician employees, are fiduciary acts within the meaning of ERISA. The Court recognized that in many cases the treatment decision and the eligibility decision (about benefits) are "inextricably mixed." For example, the eligibility decision whether to pay for emergency care often depends on a medical judgment of whether a patient's condition requires it. Similarly, whether a patient is covered for hospital care may depend on whether the medical condition requires inpatient services or can be treated adequately on an outpatient basis.[12] The Court also observed that "no HMO organization could survive without some incentive connecting physician reward with treatment rationing."

In a thoughtful article,[13] Mariner noted that although this Supreme Court decision means that managed-care organizations cannot be held directly liable as fiduciaries of ERISA plans for wrongful conduct in making "mixed" decisions about "using diagnostic tests, seeking consultations, making referrals outside the HMO network, proper standards of care, the experimental character or reasonableness of proposed therapy and whether a medical condition constitutes an emergency," it did not address the issue of federal ERISA preemption of ordinary state negligence law. Indeed, the decision could be read as implicitly agreeing with some lower-court rulings that ERISA does not preempt state court claims against managed-care plans and administrators for deliberate or negligent wrongdoing.

Without liability for wrongdoing, ERISA plans have a financial incentive to deny care. As the law is currently interpreted, at worst they will be obliged to pay only the cost of a denied benefit. "Ultimately, Congress must decide whether to preserve or eliminate the exception it has given to ERISA plans from the general rule of legal liability. One option is to amend the law to permit plan members of sue HMOs for negligence in making all types of decisions—decisions regarding eligibility, medical decisions, and mixed decisions—in state court. This would allow all claims arising from the same problem to be heard together ... [but] would undermine the goal of uniform administration of benefits" among the various states. As an alternative, the law could be changed "to allow all claims against ERISA plans and managed-care organizations to be heard in federal court and to provide the same types of compensation that are available to plaintiffs in malpractice cases in state courts, including payment for medical expenses and lost wages." This strategy would be consistent with the uniform administration of benefit plans, but could flood federal courts with unwanted claims under state common law. A third approach would be "to codify the trend in the lower courts of allowing claims under state law for negligence in making medical judgments and mixed decisions, while reserving claims regarding denial of benefits and improper administration for federal courts to decide under ERISA." However, splitting one incident into two or more different claims to be pursued in different courts would increase the time and expense of litigation. Mariner concludes that the best solution may be to overhaul the entire concept of ERISA—to establish "a separate federal statute and agency to set minimum uniform standards for *all* health plans ... [and then] delegate authority to state agencies to enforce basic administrative requirements and to state courts to hear all claims of liability." As of this date, however, all Congressional efforts to pass a "patients' bill of rights" that would eliminate the immunity of ERISA plans have been unsuccessful.

Impact on Radiologists[14]

Since ERISA health plans have been effectively immunized from medical malpractice litigation, "member employees and their beneficiaries who believe they have been injured by the medical care delivered as part of their health benefits have had, and continue to have, no choice other than to file a malpractice lawsuit against the physicians who provided the medical care rather than the insurance company or managed-care organization that may have initiated the policies that limit care." This has resulted in radiologists and other physicians subject to the strict limitations imposed by managed-care organizations being exposed to increased legal liability. Most physicians have supported the elimination of ERISA immunity in the hope that it may reduce malpractice exposure, but this might not actually be the case. As Berlin has written, plaintiffs' attorneys may not eliminate physicians as codefendants if there is a reasonable chance of finding them liable despite having the managed-care organization as a "deeper pocket." Moreover, "if HMOs become legally accountable, they may in turn attempt to exert more control over the practices of radiologists and other physicians."

It is important that a radiologist always be an advocate for his or her patient, keeping the patient's interests ahead of those of the managed care organization. As a California court observed,[15] "It is essential that cost limitation programs not be permitted to corrupt medical judgment.... A physician who complies without protest with limitations imposed by a third-party payer, when his medical judgment dictates otherwise, cannot avoid his ultimate responsibility for his patient's care." Consequently, radiologists should vigorously challenge a medical health plan if it denies or delays authorization of medically indicated diagnostic and therapeutic procedures.

Whenever possible, radiologists should refuse to sign a contract that contains a "hold harmless" clause that relieves a managed-care organization of liability for any injuries sustained by patients. Instead, radiologists should make every effort to substitute a mutual hold harmless provision, in which each party is separately responsible for its own potential liability.

Endnotes

1 Mariner WK. What recourse? Liability for managed-care decisions and the employee retirement income security act. *N Engl J Med* 2000;343:592–596.

2 Berlin L. ERISA. *AJR* 2000;174:19–25.

3 Mariner WK. What recourse? Liability for managed-care decisions and the employee retirement income security act. *N Engl J Med* 2000;343:592–596.

4 Berlin L. ERISA. *AJR* 2000;174:19–25.

5 Mariner WK. What recourse? Liability for managed-care decisions and the employee retirement income security act. *N Engl J Med* 2000;343:592–596.

6 *Dukes v U.S. Healthcare, Inc.*, 57 F2d 250 (3rd Cir 1995).

7 Mariner WK. What recourse? Liability for managed-care decisions and the employee retirement income security act. *N Engl J Med* 2000;343:592–596.

8 Berlin L. ERISA. *AJR* 2000;174:19–25.

9 *Jones v Chicago HMO Ltd. of Illinois*, 703 NE2d 502 (Ill App 1998).

10 Mariner WK. What recourse? Liability for managed-care decisions and the employee retirement income security act. *N Engl J Med* 2000;343:592–596.

11 *Pegram v Herdrich*, 2000 U.S. LEXIS 3964.

12 Mariner WK. What recourse? Liability for managed-care decisions and the employee retirement income security act. *N Engl J Med* 2000;343:592–596.

13 Ibid.

14 Berlin L. ERISA. *AJR* 2000;174:19–25.

15 *Wickline v State of California*, 192 3d 1630 (Cal App 1986).

Index